Gu

The practical v ᴊ

Your search for a weight loss book ends here!

Guilt Free

GUILT FREE BY ARUN RAO

ISBN: 9798358125476
IMPRINT: INDEPENDENTLY PUBLISHED

COMMENTS FROM MY STUDENTS AND
EARLY READERS:

The course and the book were an eye opener. We take our body, food and lifestyle for granted and never realise how important it is to balance. I tried multiple diets and failed. Methods taught by Arun are easy understand and implement. I finally found what I have been always searching for.

David G – UK

Slowly yet steadily I have lost weight. I lost nearly 14 kgs in eight months (from 95 kgs to 81 kgs). The best part, I am not gaining my weight back 😊 I strongly recommend this book to anyone who has tried many diets/ exercises and failed.

Poonam A - India

This book is about long-term weight loss, not a magic solution. It expects you to practice and try out what you're reading. I especially appreciate the writing style which is easy to understand/digest. There is no ambiguity. My summary of the book is educational, myth-busting, and weight loss without tears. I would recommend this book to anyone who does not want to spend their entire life attempting to lose weight.

Marcos T - Spain

Contents

foreword

Poem by Margaret Walker;
The women who raised me *were strong*.
They moved with the ploughs and worked hard.

They went from field to field and planted *seeds*.
When their feet *touched* the ground, the *grain grew*.
They were strong *and* liked to sing.

The women who raised me *were strong*.
My grandmothers have lots of stories to tell.

Soap, onions, and wet clay were all I could smell.
With rough veins in fast-moving hands,
They have a lot of good things to say.
The women who raised me were strong.
Why can't I be like them?

People used to stay healthy by following widely
accepted practices that were based on tribal knowledge
and lore that were passed down from generation to
generation. Health and fitness were natural and not
written. Diet, nutrition, and losing weight are not new
ideas, though. They have been around for hundreds of
years. "You are what you eat" is an old saying that has
been around for a long time. Teachings from India's
oldest books (like the yoga sutras of Patanjali, the
Bhagwad Gita, and the Upanishads) stress repeatedly
that a balanced life is the only way to live a healthy and

1

happy life. In one verse of the Bhagwad Gita, it says, "the one who eats and moves in a balanced way, does the right thing, sleeps and wakes up at regular times, and follows the path of meditation is the destroyer of pain or sadness." This message is still important and makes sense. The key message is moderation, which means to eat, sleep, work out, and do everything else in moderation.

Health and fitness are a growing business that is growing quickly every year. With obesity on the rise, being sedentary becoming the new normal, and there being no end to the number of people who want to try out new things, it will grow by a factor of 10 in the coming years and decades.

We like quick fixes and shortcuts, and there's a diet for every season. We want to lose the fat we've gained over years (or even decades) in 45 days, without giving a second thought to how bad it might be for us. Problem is, we are not designed to lose weight in 45 days. Fat gain and fat loss are both slow, which goes against what you might typically think.

Why? One argument is that the bodies we inherit through thousands and millions of years evolution is not made for sitting around all day or eating a lot of highly processed foods or sugar, the world has changed quickly, but our bodies and minds haven't caught up. Food was scarce, for most of human history, and people had to work hard to find, store, and gather food and use it during scarcity. Our bodies had to come up with clever ways to store energy and food so that we could use it when food was scarce. Strangely, if sugar and carb are bad for us, why are our minds set up to make us feel good when we eat them? Our body is a machine for survival, and our mind will do anything to keep us safe, and make sure our species lives and grows.

Our bodies and minds didn't have enough time to adapt to our current lifestyles, where we spend most of our time in front of a desk, eat processed food, crony capitalists and the political system pump more sugar into our systems. As a result, the survival mechanism that our bodies evolved is turning out to be our enemy. Even though this theory is convincing, it is too simple and far from the truth. Genes, hormones, gut microbiome (the bacteria in your gut), and the environment have all played a huge role in where we are today. We'll talk about it later.

What do you do? You join a gym for a year, but it's hard for you to even make it through a few months, hire a nutritionist and get personalised recipes? The problem is that you have to cook it yourself; and the nutritionist hasn't even tried her recipe! Try fad diets and buy a box of protein powder. Yes, we have tried it all and failed repeatedly. Well, the easiest and cheapest thing to do (and I'm sure you've done it many times) is to make a birthday or new year's resolution, I could say a lot more.

I confess, I have done it all, I have struggled with my weight my whole life. My mother says that when I was born, I was heavier than the average healthy child. No one knew I had a natural tendency to gain weight quickly and that my average weight was always on the edge. Even though I was heavier than most of my friends, I was never obese. My body knew and had found a "sweet spot" where my weight went up and down but never made the scale tip. Ask my family and friends, they know the only unchanging thing about me is my weight. In my teens, I realized that my asthma is linked to my weight. I also noticed that the "sweet spot" kept getting bigger over the years because my body kept setting the bar higher without me knowing. I used to have more asthma attacks when I was heavier. Even worse, because I had exercise-induced asthma, exercise made my asthma attacks worse, as soon my weight went down, so did my bouts and even the ones that were caused by exercise stopped. My wake-up call happened when I was 18 years old, from that day on, I've been on a collision course with my weight for 23 years.

I've read all the best-selling books (though only a few of them were good), tried many diets (you name it, I've tried it), failed many times, and experimented on my body. The problem with the books – none of them gave me a complete picture. They often ended up confusing me and my journey always ended in disappointment.

Eventually, I was able to find light at the end of the tunnel, I've been at the right weight for over a decade and a half now, and I've kept it that way through many changes and improvements.

If you're still concerned about credentials. I'm a trained nutritionist, but the course was useless to me because it was so disconnected from reality. For the past few years, I have taught weekend offline weight management course and I am transitioning to a weekend online model. Many of my students have noticed tangible effects and this motivated me to write the book; I used the same template that I used for my course for this book. I am however limited by the number of pages in this book when compared with the course.

If you are more interested in the online course, please contact me here[1](see end of chapter 9). I also intend to build a YouTube channel where you may find excerpts from the course I have conducted in the past; please stay tuned to my WhatsApp and email subscriber lists[2] (see end of chapter 9) for regular updates.

I'm however not an expert on diets, or a fitness trainer, and I don't have a six-pack or big muscles. I have fought with my weight my whole life. I walk and run, and I can put you to the test. I have worked hard for 23 years to live a healthy life and keep my mind healthy. I have also trained hundreds of students in India over the past few years.

Physically and even more so mentally, it is hard to lose weight and keep it off. I can see why you chose this book and have read so far, and I'd like to help you. Don't you agree that there are many ways to get wise and find yourself a way out?

I know the look you're giving; this guy is not an expert

on fitness. He hasn't worked with celebrities. What can he do for me? Before you judge me, I'd like to know how long your grandparents and great-grandparents lived. And did they ever go to a nutritionist, gym, or fitness expert? How did they live long, happy, and healthy lives? The answer is that they learned from the mistakes of many people before them and inculcated the same in their everyday lifestyle. They cracked the code without even realising it, while we couldn't figure it out.

There is too much information, people are confused and have lost touch with the real world. We don't know the right from wrong because everyone seems to be right. People in their 30s and 40s are dying of heart problems. Even people who go to the gym and are otherwise fit are dying, leaving doctors to scratch their heads. You can put your body at risk and join the crowd, or you can use the wisdom that our ancestors used and find a permanent cure. Choice is yours.

In the 20th century, we have used health and weight as if they were the same thing. This is because both the media and the medical industry have been so focused on weight and fat. You don't have to be skinny to be healthy. Having the right weight is only one part of being healthy. The obsession with losing weight has made people feel bad about their bodies. Were your grandmothers skinny? You may have noticed that some of your family or friends have fat deposits but still live a healthy and long life. On the other end of the spectrum, we have seen healthy-looking people go through bouts of depression, have a negative body image, are never happy with their weight, are always trying to lose weight, and are otherwise unhealthy. Did you know that smokers typically weigh less than non-smokers? Does it mean that they are healthy? (Read chapter Mind I control you). Unfortunately, our body weight is not a good indicator of how healthy we are.

There is too much information; media, health, food, and maybe even the pharmaceutical industries all have a vested interest in making us feel bad and paranoid. For example, the US weight loss industry is well over $70 billion. Why do people have such a high stake? The more worried you are, the more likely it is that you will buy fat free milk, a protein bar, a weight loss pill, join a gym, or take part in a weight loss programme only to gain all the weight they lost in 45 days after the programme.

You don't need a protein bar or protein shake; we don't need a weight loss pill, you don't need to go to the gym and pump your muscles or join a weight loss programme. Any small weight loss benefits you might get come at the cost of your health, and the benefits will wear off quickly, leaving you back at square one. They market easy weight loss solution with no explanation and little investigation.

Research has shown that people who do things to control their weight end up having trouble with their weight because they were focused on their weight and not their general health. In the long run, your health is more important than how much you weigh. Yes, it's important to be a certain weight and not have a lot of visceral fat, which is the fat around your organs. But weight shouldn't be the end goal. If you are obsessed with losing weight, you might do things that are bad for you, like go on a diet, join a fast weight loss programme, work out until you die, or use so-called weight loss products that do more harm than good.

We don't realise that our weight changes over time; we gain and lose weight over time, our weight changes naturally depending on the season, food we eat, and our body type etc. Weight loss is a complicated process and depends on a combination of factors. Diets and exercise cannot achieve weight loss.

This book with teach you to stop obsessing over your weight and start focusing on healthy habits; like making the right food choices and keeping your emotions in check. It will also teach you that exercise isn't a way to lose weight, but just something you have to do for your overall health. What you need to do right now is throw away the scale.

This book is a collection of all the lessons I've learned over the years. Even though I tried to organise the content in a logical and sequential way, you could pick any chapter at random and it would still make sense.

You could also easily connect one topic to another.

Guilt Free will bring you back to earth. It is not one more book about a fad diet. It doesn't give you fancy recipes. Instead, it helps you balance your diet as much as possible by giving you tips on how to get the most out of the food your mom or grandma used to cook. You already know that fad diets only work for a short time. You lose weight, but then you gain it all back. Most fad diets hurt you more than they help. The problem with diet plans and recipes is that they don't work in the long run. Our minds are used to the foods we ate when we were young, and they will resist any change. People are social creatures, we don't like to stand out in a crowd, so we try to blend in the crowd. People celebrate, and sweets are a symbol of and a part of celebration, we have also made up many reasons to celebrate and eat sweets throughout the year. It takes a lot of self-control to stick to a diet every day.

Will power and human creativity are strange things to put together. Our clever mind will trick itself and give us a false sense of control. We'll change the diet programme to make it fit our needs, which throws off the nutrition balance that dieticians work hard to achieve. And before you knew it, the diet has failed. In the long run, all diets that try to keep track of calories and nutrients will fail. Your brain and body behave as if they don't care about your weight or your weight-loss aim, and they don't care how you look.

Guilt Free doesn't send you to the gym every day or suggest that you join a weight loss programme. The advice I've given is easy to understand and put into action. Even our hunter-gatherer ancestors never worked out, they spent most of their time sitting when they weren't hunting or gathering, the only time they really moved their bodies was when they were hunting, gathering, or for recreation (like a dance). We don't have a natural drive to work out or run if we're not doing it for fun (like a dance) or to find food and this is the reason, it's hard to get up and work out every day. (Chapter 06 has More on this).

Guilt Free will help you understand why your body does what it does. It doesn't stigmatise being fat, it will teach you the oldest and most reliable way to lose weight and keep it off. It will help you learn how to be happy with yourself. It will give you the tools you need to write your code for losing weight. Your search for a book to help you lose weight is over.

People may say that this book doesn't say much about meat, which I admit is partially true. I'm not in favour of any diet (vegetarian or non-vegetarian). I was born into a strict vegetarian family, and for the first 20 years of my life, I ate only plant-based food. I changed my mind and I ate meat for the next five years. But in the last ten years, I stopped eating meat and turned into a vegetarian. Even though I have my own reasons for being a vegetarian and a vegan, I am not a firm supporter of veganism. I'd actually tell someone to keep eating the way their grandparents did (be it vegetarian or non-vegetarian). Meat is easy to get because meat production is now industrialised and more restaurants serving meat are opening up all around us. But it's important to remember that humans can't get their energy from meat alone. People need to eat carbs to get energy, and carb is the reason we gain weight, not because of meat. This book is mostly about carbs, which people have always gotten from plants and trees. I've had a few friends who were adamantly against eating fruits and vegetables and didn't want to eat them at all. I don't agree with this philosophy, because I think that everyone, vegetarian or not, needs to eat fruits and vegetables as part of a healthy diet. People have changed over time to become omnivores instead of just carnivores. Our bodies, digestive systems, and evolutionary history show that we can live on both meat and plant-based foods (most of the time cooked meat). Even 100–200 years ago, it was harder for our ancestors to get meat than it is for us today. Some research shows that as much as 70% of a hunter gatherer's diet comprised plants, since gathering food was much easier than hunting. Forest tribes still don't get to hunt every day, and hunters often come back empty-handed. We don't seem to have grown to live off of meat alone. There is also conclusive evidence that we could not have lived off of meat alone or that we mostly ate plant-based foods. Even though research has shown that eating a lot of meat (especially processed meat) can be bad in other ways, it does not cause weight gain.

I really want to help and support you. I don't want to write just to make a few dollars and then leave. If you don't like what's in the book or don't think it was worth your hard-earned money, you don't have to buy it. I promise to give you all of your money back, no questions asked, if you are not happy with the content or methods. Just get in touch with me, and I'll give you the money back.

Chapter 1

Myth Buster: The truth is right there in plain sight

Chapter 1 - Myth Buster: The truth is right there in plain sight

I agree you know a few things about food, diets, losing weight, and living a healthy life. I used to think the same way. But my beliefs and lessons have often been wrong. Maybe you only chose this book because you thought it would differ from others. Even I've had a hard time, though, because I've tried everything, read many books, subscribed to gym many times, tried many diets.

Here goes a saying in Sanskrit

"It is easy to make a fool happy. A wise man is easier to convince. But even the creator can't convince a self-important snob who brags about how much he knows."

The saying fits our lives beautifully. I'm not putting down your knowledge or trying to discourage you. All I'm saying is that we never stop learning, and we always learn from our mistakes.

My goal is to help you get through this. My job is hard because I'm not trying to teach an ignorant man (or woman), and I don't think we're one of the few smart people. It's dangerous to only know half of something.

In the following chapters, we would end up busting a few myths and figuring out how our bodies and minds work, as well as how to make slight changes in our lifestyle and get enormous benefits. Even though a lot of what I'm writing might seem obvious, we often over-index and take things for granted. It's time to stop, turn around, look again, learn something new, let go of old habits and ideas, make slight changes, and build a better version of yourself.

Here are a few myths that this book busts.

Myth 1: Dangerous carbohydrate:

Carbohydrates, or carbs, are often bad-mouthed by people who recommend trendy diets, but they are still an important part of our diet because they give us the fuel we need. Carbs give the body and the nervous system energy. If you don't get enough of this important macronutrient, it could hurt your body and mind. Carbs are not dangerous because they are the building blocks of our bodies and we need them to live. What's important is what carbs you eat (processed or natural).

For example, an adult human brain at rest uses up about 20–25% of the glucose that the whole body needs at rest. Even though the brain only makes up 2% of the body's weight, it uses about 25% of the body's energy. Glucose, also called "carbs" is the primary fuel for the brain.

2. Diets work: (low carb, high fat, and high protein)

In a single Google search, you may find various websites and blogs with countless diet regimens, recipes, and other weight loss aids. However, there are many factors beyond hunger, self-control, and dietary restrictions that influence how much and what kinds of food you eat.

Diets don't work. We've all tried one diet or another that didn't work, but that's a fact. Why does it fail? Maybe we've been asking the wrong question. All the diet books have tried to find a diet that works for everyone.

The diets don't consider things like the food our ancestors had for thousands of years (the diet that helped our grandparents live and thrive), our genetic makeup and predispositions, our hormonal predispositions, our gut microbiome, and our way of life. Any diet that doesn't take these things into account will fail. I was part of a core family of over 30 people for many years. We all lived and ate together. We almost always ate the same things every day. Still, one or two of my cousins were heavier than the rest, and a few of them were slimmer. Initially, I couldn't figure out how the same diet could make different people react in different ways.

The answer to this question could be that the effects of diet depend on the person and as a corollary, if we customize the existing diet to a person's make-up, it works.

We've been looking for an egg everywhere, even though we have a chicken in our backyard. Our ancestors had already come up with tried and tested diet that was made to fit each person's body type. Our forefathers diet worked perfectly well for generations and they survived on this diet for ages without a single problem the current generation is facing. Their diet was wholesome, had variety, tasted better and yet obesity was never a problem.

For example, in India, rice is the staple food in over 20 States in the south, east, and northeast, while wheat is the staple food in the north and west (i.e., the Hindi heartland). People who eat rice, consume wheat occasionally and people in north India eat rice occasionally. New research shows that a person's glucose/insulin response to a certain food can be very different depending on their genes, hormones, and other factors. So, a dietary guideline that is made for everyone will fail. In fact, the first thing a dietitian would tell someone is to stop eating rice. They don't think for a second that rice is a staple food for over three billion people around the world. Do you see three billion obese people in Asia? Asians have been eating rice-based meals for thousands of years and many generations. Asians have been healthy for a long time by eating rice, vegetables, meat, and fruit. Diet is attractive and promises quick solution, we get sucked into it repeatedly without looking at the broader picture.

Problem is, we no longer eat the way our ancestors did because of lack of time and western food. And this is the problem with the diet books. You can't prescribe the same diet for everyone. We should make a diet that fit the needs of each person. All that was needed was to tweak the diets we already had and make them work best for our bodies.

Diets that are low in carbs, high in protein, and high in fat are often talked about by weight loss experts. Some diets that come to mind are Atkins Diet, the Paleo diet, the Keto Diet, etc. These and more are often called the Ketogenic diet. Some of these diets depend on limiting carbs and making up for them with healthy fats and protein. Fats should make up as much as 90% of your daily calorie intake. On a typical Keto diet, a person eats between 150 and 175 gms of fat, 40 to 50 gms of Carbs, and 75 gms of protein every day. The exact ratio keeps varying though. All of this seems great and interesting because people are giving you a recipe for weight loss that you might follow. The problem is that people are jumping on the bandwagon without thinking about how it might hurt them. Firstly, I'm sure you agree with me that the diet changes how our bodies react. Our bodies have a delicate balance of the nutrients they need, and they have ways to find, store, and get rid of them. How our body processes food is still largely unknown because it depends on things like our age, gender, metabolism, genes, lifestyle, processed food in the diet, season, our mental state etc. whereas dieting does not view these aspects holistically.

Here are some health risks that could come from the keto low-carb diets:

Nutrition: How do you get the right amount of nutrition and deal with the risks of not getting enough? How sure are we that everyone will stick to the diet to the letter? The problem with rule books is that people always want to change, twist, and adapt to them. You already know what can happen when you don't get enough nutrition. Can you guarantee a healthy and balanced diet?

Internal organs: Our internal organs are designed to process a balanced diet, any change that lasts for a long time will influence the internal organs.

Effects on mood—We already knew this about people who had tried Keto or were on a low carb diet. As was already said, our brains need carbohydrates to work well and stay healthy. If you don't give the brain food that comes easily and naturally, it will have to get its energy from stored energy, which will cause mood swings and make you angry.

Do you know what made the Keto diet popular and

how it started? During their research, scientists found that the children with epilepsy who were put on Keto diet had fewer epileptic seizures. This was not a weight loss tool originally!

Also, it's important to remember that research on the topic is still going on, and I couldn't find any credible scientific data (tested on a fairly large sample population) on how the Keto diet works. If you still think Keto is the right diet for you, please get advice from someone with a solid background.

Not convinced? Let's talk about leptin; leptin is a satiety hormone that aids in weight regulation and has recently attracted a lot of attention, as it might aid in weight management. Leptin is found in fat cells and is released in response to changes in energy balance and fat mass.

Hypothalamus (our brain's "eating control center") is alerted when leptin is released; the hypothalamus then helps change regulatory signals (i.e., fullness cues) that help to reset our fat and energy levels.

People with unhealthy, high weights are thought to be leptin resistant. Leptin resistance occurs when fat cells cannot respond to changes in energy and fat mass. As a result, they may miss fullness signs even when their bodies have enough energy[3] where they end up consuming more energy than required.

Weight management is not simple. The orchestration of how our bodies manage weight is extremely deep. For example, evidence reveals that leptin does more than only keep us from overeating. Instead, it could be biased to keep our bodies from losing fat rather than growing fat. Leptin's principal function may be to keep us from going below our set-point weight, with less concern about weight gain. No wonder it is easier to have set weight or even gain, but difficult to lose it.

Further, sustained calorie restriction diet over a long period is difficult. The habenula is a small area in the centre of the brain, between the thalamus and the pineal gland stalk. We also known it as the "Anti-reward system." It has a significant impact on how the brain perceives pleasure, pain, worry, and tension. The habenula regulates surrounding reward zones and assists us in learning from our actions in life. It is the motivation switch for your weight loss quest.

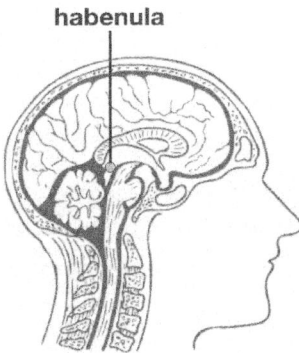

Image credit - https://www.brainpost.co

Setting a precise weight loss goal or outcome can be difficult because if you don't achieve it, your habenula urges you to quit trying, even if things are not going well.

Habenula awakens when your diet doesn't give you the desired result, such as expecting to lose a pound within a week and ending up losing nothing or gaining back lost weight.

You then become obsessed with tracking calories, carbs, or steps, and you lose sight of what is truly important. You've been reprogrammed to prioritize rewards over goals. The goal is to lead a healthy life, we lose sight of the goal and get obsessed with calorie and tracking steps/ miles.

When you do not receive the desired reward, your lateral habenula becomes aroused and dampens your motivation to attempt again. The more frequently this cycle occurs, the easier it is for your lateral habenula to activate and stop it.

Things grow alarming when the habenula transmits signals at the wrong times. It may cause you to give up before you even begin, where it triggers negative self-talk. Habenula works as a kill switch, making you not want to try that diet again.

Another cause of habenula is that your body opposes restrictive diets and that your brain regulates your body weight. When you go on a restrictive diet, stress hormones are released, and ignoring your hunger all the time makes it difficult to make smart selections and maintain your weight.

Your body has a predetermined weight that is unrelated to how you appear or how much weight you wish to reduce. The hormones ghrelin and leptin keep your body's set point constant. They signal to your body when you're hungry or full. If significant changes in your diet or lifestyle result in drastic weight reduction, these hormones detect an imbalance and go on an overdrive, your brain will force you to perform activities you know are comfortable (such as eating energy dense foods or junk) in order to return you to your set position.

Therefore, the brain frequently makes losing weight difficult. Weeks of eating calorie restricted food suddenly collapses with a single demotivating event. Habenula will see this as a failure and make you less likely to try again on your weight-loss journey. The intention is to protect you, yet all it accomplishes is to make you less likely to attempt again. The reward pathway instructs you to perform something pleasurable in order to cope with the stress.

Let me repeat, diets don't work. Our body and mind are complex machinery, don't take a simplistic approach. Don't just pick up a diet book and start dieting. Talk to your doctor first. Otherwise, you're putting your body in danger and giving the author more money from royalties. Please don't rely on rumours or stories about how someone's friend tried a diet, and it worked for them, etc.

It is important to consult a specialist (your family doctor) before you actually start a diet.

Myth 2: Calories are bad for you

That you should eat less and move more has been around for a long time. People think that if you eat fewer calories than you need to burn, you will create a "calorie deficit," which will force your body to burn fat to make up for it. This will cause you to lose weight (simple math: calorie deficit + exercise = weight loss), the easiest way to lose weight is to eat less than you burn.

You can pick any packaged food and it will tell you how many calories you should eat each day, and it will compare the food to this guideline. And the government has made rules about how many calories an adult man or woman should eat each day. How the heck do they think we can tell in a second if something is healthy or not just by looking at the label? I mean, do you know how many calories you are consuming otherwise during the day? How are we to do the math in our heads and conclude? They added fat to the mix to rub salt in the wound. Most of the time, the label has confused me and not helped me at all.

There is a lot of information out there about calories, and when you get on a treadmill, it counts the calories you burn. There are apps and Fitness trackers that can help you keep track of calories.

Calories are so common that they are written on all labels around the world. You can't get away from the calorie curse, even if you want to. I still don't understand why putting calories on the label is a good idea or how it changes people's decisions.

Counting calories, cutting back on calories, and burning calories has always been the most important part of any plan of losing weight.

What is a calorie, by the way? A calorie is a unit that tells how much energy a food or drink has. It is not something that is in the food you eat. Instead, it is a way to measure how much energy the food gives off after you eat it. Calorie only measures the amount of energy and not the amount or type of nutrients. Calories are neither our friends nor are they our enemies. They let us compare the amount of energy in one type of food to another.

Even though the number of calories is always the same, how our bodies process calories can be very different, depending on things like hormone levels, genetics, and basic metabolic rates to name a few. Because of this, our bodies will process and burn calories in different ways. For example, two people who weigh the same will need different amounts of calories.

The problem with counting calories is that we look at the body simply, like a car; just like you measure a car's mileage, we measure a person's calorific needs. The Problem is that we don't have software built into hardware (like a robot) that can calculate how many calories a person needs. Our bodies are not machines, we are living beings that have changed over millions or billions of years; genes, hormones, enzymes, the environment, and other things work together in a complicated way to make up our bodies. Cutting calories doesn't make you healthier, and there's no proof that counting and limiting calories makes you healthier or helps you lose weight in the long run. It might only last for a short time. The question is whether it will help you stay healthy? You know the answer already. Even if you lose weight in the short term, it will stop going down and come back with a bang in the long term.

People who like diets always say that cutting calories and working out is the magic pill. Still, the devil is in the details. I have found that the weight loss doesn't always happen in a way that makes sense or is proportional.

One reason, is eating right after working out. My body and mind have naturally made me hungrier on days I work out, where I trick myself by telling that "one cookie is okay today because I worked out." There is a lot of mental chatter and a strong desire to make up for it. I have noticed that when I work out, I eat more calories than when I don't. This is so natural that I notice my five-year-old son eating more on days when he has physical education at school. I'm sure you or someone else has a similar personal story. For example, one thing that has always puzzled me is when a friend or family member eats a lot but stays about the same weight. On the other end of the spectrum, a friend who eats moderately but still gains weight. You don't have to look too far. Even if two people in the same family eat the same food, their fat profiles will be different. People somehow keep their average weight and don't gain a lot of weight quickly, which you might think they would do based on and their calorie intake. What is going on? They eat more calories than most people, but don't get fatter? The simple answer is that their body is trying to stay in its sweet spot by burning more calories.

The mechanism of how our bodies determine burning calories, storing fat are complex and still unknown. However, Set-point theory[4] says that each person has a biologically predetermined weight (Sweet spot) where their body works best. So, each person's body works to keep them at their sweet spot by adjusting different biological systems. This helps regulate how much food a person eats and how much energy they use.

Set-point theory helps explain why many people gain back weight they've lost. It also explains why people with eating disorders aren't always very thin, our bodies fight to keep us at or above our set-point weights.

Here is where the theory of a "calorie deficit" falls apart. It doesn't consider how a person's body works.

But I have also noticed that the set point is slowly but steadily set higher in people who gain weight although the body will try to burn more calories to stay in the sweet spot. But as your hormones change, the sweet spot moves up ever so slightly, and you are on a slippery slope to weight gain without even realising it. The calorie deficit hypothesis is being disproven by ton of scientific writing and research and yet we force ourselves to believe the theory.

There is no one size that fits all, no common yardstick that we could all use as a standard. The biggest loser is an American TV show in which overweight people compete against each other and end up losing a lot of weight. it will make you wonder how they changed so much. Think they sustained their weight loss? Why don't you just look it up on google?

The potential risk of cutting calories:

Remember that you can't control how your body uses the calories you eat because they come from the outside. Your body will think it is starving and stop burning fat. Instead, it will use up your stored protein. Why? Relatively, protein is easier to burn when compared with fat and your body wants to conserve fat. Even though you might lose weight temporarily, most people feel weak and gain weight in the long run. Also, a common misconception is that you can lose weight by cutting back on calories and working out. Well, think about this, when you cut back on calories and work out, you will get tired quickly because your body is in a "conservation mode" and wants to save fat whenever it can. The only way for your body to save energy is to use less of it. The body is a great example of how evolution works. You have little control over it, and it will do anything to help you stay alive, even temporarily shutting you down. The body will try to find the path with the least resistance, and it will push you toward a state of balance where it will do its best to help you gain back the weight you lost. Who will win the fight between the body and the mind? You can guess just as well as I can.

Mood and brain: Cutting calories will mess up your brain, your hormones, and willpower. You think about food all the time. Because your brain is getting less glucose, you get brain fog, mood swings, irritability, lethargy, trouble focusing, etc., and before you know it, you end up bingeing!

The symptom–The problem is not the number of calories in food. The problem is biological.

Clearly, cutting calories is not a good long-term solution. The Problem is that eating fewer calories doesn't have a long-term effect, and when the tables turn and you can't keep it up, social stigma (people will say, "See, I told you! "), self-loathing, and resentment will set in, and things will go downhill from there. Anyone who has tried a low-calorie diet will agree with this.

"It takes a wise man to learn from his own mistakes, but an even wiser man to learn from others," says a Zen proverb.

We know the calorie restriction theory is not true. We know that people who recommend to cut calories are taking us for a ride, but few see or listen. Why is counting calories so common, and how did people start doing it? Maybe its beauty comes from how easy it is to do. If we know that a slice of bread has 100 calories, a chocolate chip cookie has 60 calories, a slice of pizza has 200 calories, and so on, it's easy to make a mental map of calories. Our minds are may be made to take shortcuts and keeping things simple, makes it easier to count calories.

Myth 3: It's all in the genes.

Yes, there is a clear link between genes and weight gain. As you will learn in later chapters, blaming weight gain on diet or overeating alone is a mistake. Overeating and gaining weight may just be symptoms, and the real problem may be a mix of nature (our genes) and nurture (the way we have tuned our hormonal mechanisms over many decades or many years for young people). It's a pessimistic way to think to think that our genes make us fat and that we may have to live with the risks that come with being overweight. Yes, we can lose weight and still be healthy. The first step to getting there is to change the "nurture," so we have to unlearn many beliefs and habits, take the right steps, and keep going, even if we have short-term setbacks. Slowly but surely, you will see changes in nature too (perhaps at an epigenetic level). Let's not give up on our lives. Instead, let's think positively and keep telling our brains positive things. Eventually, this will lead to action and actual results.

Myth 4: We get fat when we eat too much.

Overeating is a sign of weight gain, not the reason people gain weight. Few studies have overfed people on purpose to find out what happens when you eat too much. Strangely, few of the people gave up because they just couldn't eat enough. Some people's bodies burned more calories than they took in because they were trying hard to stay in the "sweet spot."

We gain weight over long periods of time (decades) for several reasons. We can't just starve ourselves to lose weight. There are clear hormonal pathways in our bodies that tell us when we are hungry and when we are full. Hormones cause weight gain. As soon as we figure out how hormones work, we lose weight. There are some exceptions, though. People eat more than usual when they eat ultra-processed food because processed food has many times as much energy per volume and weight as unprocessed food. For example, a glass of orange juice has the same amount of fructose as 6 and 8 oranges. You can drink a glass of orange juice in one gulp, but can you eat eight oranges at once?

Maybe people have gained weight not because they eat too much, but because they depend on highly processed foods.

Myth 5: Sugar substitutes

There is no good reason to use Artificial sweeteners. They hurt our bodies in ways that are bad. There is no such thing as a good, bad, natural, or unnatural sugar substitute. All sugar substitutes are bad.

Myth 6–Exercise overdrive

To lose weight, we pull our socks up, make a new year or birthday resolution to shed the extra pounds, we subscribe to a gym membership and diligently start a regimen. Physical activity is undeniably good for you (see chapter 06); however, exercise to lose weight will surely backfire.

For starters, studies[5] have shown that typically recommended exercise regime of 30 mins moderate to intense exercise has little weight loss effect. Naysayers will then say exercise should be combined with calorie restriction to produce tangible results. Well, this[6] study has shown that calorie restriction, along with exercise, shows modest weight loss in the subjects where the weight plateaus after 6 months. Subjects could maintain their weight but not drastically reduce it. This[7] study, however, demonstrated that high-intensity exercise results in weight loss; however, the amount of exercise required to achieve this weight loss was significantly higher than the overall guidelines for healthy exercise (i.e., 30 mins).

I used to work out for 90–120 minutes every day, five days a week. I used to think that I could lose weight by working out. When we work out, our bodies don't get enough glucose, so instead of burning stored energy (i.e., fat), our bodies will look for instant gratification, and our minds will tell us to grab something high in calories. Calorie restriction where we obsessively track and count calories and lose weight. Yes, I have noticeably lost a lot of weight in a short amount of time. However, I gained it all back and plateaued within the next few quarters. Question is, why is it difficult to lose weight by exercise alone, why don't we drastically reduce weight and why do we gain it all back? Well, there is no straightforward answer. Here are few potential explanations.

Old habits die hard and without even realising, we compensate the exercise with energy consumption. We grab a cookie or a slice of pizza. I used to think just one cookie will do no harm. Well, consider this, do 45 minutes of intense swimming to burn one slice of pizza or you should walk for 30 mins briskly to burn a small bottle of fruit juice.

We may compensate physiologically, for example, on days of exercise, I used to sit more than usual. We compensate the excessive exercise with non-activity.

Blundell et al[8]. suggested that people vary a lot in how much they exercise and how much food they eat. Our food intake is dependent on our overall fat mass (remember effect of Leptin and Leptin resistance), our resting metabolic rate, our hormonal response and other genetic predispositions. These factors vary from person to person, making it hard to predict how each person will respond to exercise and weight loss.

One of the bigger problems with exercising to lose weight is the mental burden, where exercise is no more recreational, it is more of a regimen and a burden. It is like making a child do chores.

Weight loss by exercise and calorie restriction is not sustainable and We often give up on exercise when it doesn't help us lose weight the way we thought it would (remember the Habenula effect).

The message here is that exercise and calorie restriction is perceived by our mind and body as a punishment and we are unlikely to sustain it for a long time as the body-mind-hormone-genes combination is complex and works against typical logical thinking.

The problem with exercise-induced and calorie-restricted weight loss is, we are not training our internal machinery to gradually reduce the sweet spot. Things happen all of a sudden, the body considers this out of the ordinary, although you may think you are overweight, the body thinks it is the ideal weight and it will try it's best to bring your weight back to the sweet spot.

Am I saying, physical activity is waste of time? No, physical activity should be part of overall well-being and not used as a weight-loss tool. Physical activity, should be part of a holistic solution and not the only option.

The myths that I have highlighted are indicative and not exhaustive. We will learn and unlearn many beliefs in the next few pages. Weight management is a complex topic and there is no one reason people gain weight. It is always because of a combination of factors. Our body behaves as though it has a mind of its own!

Chapter 2
The body has its own mind!

Chapter 2 - The body has its own mind!

We already know that some people put on weight more quickly than others. As I mentioned earlier, some people can burn calories more quickly than others. While some people are too sensitive and gain weight faster than others. I've also seen people stay thin until middle age, then slowly gain weight until they reach their ideal weight, as if their bodies turned on a switch when they hit middle age.

Simply put, we take in calories, burn as many as we need, and store the rest as fat. But gaining weight depends on many things that are set by genes and environment. Even though either or both can have a big effect, genes are easier to explain. Few people call it hereditary, like heart disease, mental illness, diabetes, high blood pressure, etc., that makes us more likely to gain weight. There may be hundreds of genes that cause weight gain, but only a few of them may have a big effect. Genes mess up the way our bodies work. For example, if there are underlying mental health problems, there may be slight changes in hunger, fullness, hormones, organ function, metabolism, and certain behavioral tendencies (such as bingeing during times of stress). One or more of these things could tip the scale in your favour or against you. Let's make things a little harder, even the effects of genes can differ from one person to the next. For example, a person's genes may make them so likely to be overweight that no matter what they do, they will always gain weight. In other situations, a person may fall under a median, so their genes play a small but important role and their environment and lifestyle make it worse; most people fall in this category. heavy predisposition means some people may need help from a specialist or a doctor.

Our environment, our actions, and the choices we make have subtle but long-lasting effects on us. Some changes in our bodies will cause us to gain weight without us even realising it. Obesity is getting worse among people and around the world (perhaps a steep curve). Surely, genetics are not the only reason for the alarming rise.

Environmental factors can start in the womb before a child is even born, in the way a child acts, and how a person lives in their early, middle, and later years.

For example, parents who are obese but whose own parents were not obese or overweight may pass this trait on to their children even before the child is born. Parents can teach their kids things that will make them more likely to gain weight as adults, like giving them sugary drinks, ultra-processed food, or encouraging them to be less active. Lastly, many modern lifestyle changes, like a reliance on ultra-processed food ([9],[10]) and sugar ([11],[12]), have an effect of accretion, where one thing leads to another and ends up in changes at a hormonal level, like insulin resistance. We are setting up a fat baby factory without even realising it, and this is putting the lives of the next generation at risk.

Also, because there are so many diets in the market, we go "diet shopping," which causes us to lose and gain weight in cycles. Strangely, this cycle creates a pattern and makes it more likely that you will gain weight[13].

No–You cannot lose weight and sustain by:

1. Dieting
2. Restricting calories
3. Counting calories
4. Going on a low-carb diet
5. Exercising
6. Restricting calories and exercising
7. Starving

Yes, - People gain weight for several reasons, including genes, complex hormonal interplay and neurological pathways, the environment, ultra-processed foods, sugar, lack of exercise, stress, and so on[14]. However, "insulin" is the main reason people gain weight.

Chapter 3
Insulin: boon or bane?

Chapter 3 - Insulin: boon or bane?

Let's try a thought experiment.

What happens to a healthy person's weight if I give insulin three times a day before meals?

Answer: His weight goes up.

What happens to a person's weight if the pancreas is told to stop making insulin?

Answer: The person will lose weight in a big way.

People with diabetes need insulin, in one form or another. People with diabetes who take insulin know all too well that they gain weight and have a hard time losing weight even if they try to limit calories and or work out. Also, people with type 1 diabetes make no insulin or very little insulin. This happens because antibodies kill beta cells in the pancreas. With no insulin to neutralise glucose, the blood and urine have a lot of glucose. But one of the most noticeable signs of type 1 diabetes is an unintentional weight loss.

The pancreas makes a hormone called insulin. Certain parts of the pancreas, called beta cells, make insulin and it is pumped directly into the bloodstream, where its primary job is to make sure that the body uses the carbohydrate in food in the right way.

As we saw in myth 1, carbs are still an important part of how our bodies work because they give our bodies the fuel they need. Carbs give the body and the nervous system energy.

During digestion in the intestines, the intestinal valve stretches and opens up to make room for the food.

This Causes a complex reaction in which hormones and nervous reflexes work together to control the activity of the stomach, making some gastric juices and stop others at the same time.

The intestine takes in glucose from carbohydrates and releases it into the bloodstream. This causes glucose molecules to be released into the bloodstream. When glucose levels rise, they tell the pancreas to release insulin to get the glucose out of the blood. Insulin is like a messenger that delivers a message and tells the liver, muscles, and fat to take in glucose and use it for energy. Note that cells, muscles, the liver, and other organs can't absorb glucose in its original form because insulin is needed to open the pathways for absorption. When the body works well, this process gets rid of the glucose made when carbs are devoured. This doesn't happen when there is no insulin or very little insulin, which results in raising the blood sugar levels.

HOW DOES INSULIN WORK

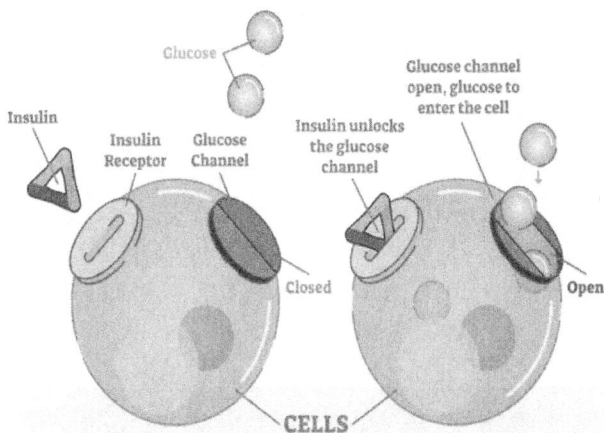

Image credit: VectorMine/Shutterstock.com

Insulin is a hormone, and its job is to control how much glucose is in the blood. It works closely with the central nervous system where it controls how much food the body eats and how much it weighs. In terms of quantum of insulin released, the amount of glucose in the blood is directly related to how much insulin is released. When the amount of glucose in the body goes down, insulin goes down too.

People who eat a lot of protein should know that even protein causes an insulin response, so protein raises the amount of insulin in the bloodstream. When you eat protein[15], your body responds by making insulin.

Insulin is needed for the body to use glucose, control, fat, and store fat. When we are eating, the amount of insulin in the blood is directly related to how many carbohydrates we eat (we will get to what happens in the fasting state in the fasting chapter).

The liver stores energy as glycogen and turns glucose into glycogen with the help of insulin. Insulin also acts as a stimulant. The liver stores glycogen so that we can use it later when there isn't enough glucose in the blood. Extra glycogen that the liver can't store is turned into fat so that it can be used later, a process called de novo lipogenesis (meaning - to make new fat). When we don't get enough glucose, like when we're sleeping and don't eat, your blood glucose level goes down. This instructs your pancreas to make glucagon a hormone. Glucagon tells your liver and muscle cells to turn the glycogen they have stored into glucose. The glucose is then sent to the rest of your cells so they can use it for energy. The insulin and glycogen interplay ensure your blood sugar does not drop too low, so that your body always has enough energy.

Then, the body moves on to stored fat, which is broken down and burned for energy (a process known as Lipolysis meaning fat breakdown). Fat has a lot of energy but is hard to break down because the body breaks down glycogen first. When our bodies can't get enough energy from glycogen, they break down fat and turn it into energy (for instance between dinner and breakfast, energy exertion etc.,).

Insulin's primary job is to send glucose to cells and store fat. Insulin has an indirect effect on fat because it tells the body to stop breaking down fat and store fat.

As soon as insulin is released, fat breakdown stops and fat build up starts.

Now, think about the person in our thought experiment. He takes insulin three times a day and might eat three or more meals a day. His body doesn't have time to break down fat, so it keeps storing it. On the other end of the spectrum is a person with type 1 diabetes. If there isn't enough insulin, glucose can't get into the cells, so glucose builds up in the blood and urine. The body needs energy, so it burns fat and muscle to get it. This leads to weight loss.

The body goes through a phase called the cephalic phase, during which it gets ready to eat or waits for food (perhaps you are sitting in a restaurant and waiting for food). During this phase, the body is getting ready to eat. The phase begins with seeing, smelling, tasting, or even just thinking about food. This phase is a conditioned response, where a complex neurological process happens depending on how you have trained your body and mind (for example, by eating dinner at 10 PM). Some estimates say that over twenty stomach juices are made at this point. Researchers [16]have shown that the body also starts making insulin and putting it into the bloodstream. Just seeing food stops fat from being broken down!

Here is where eating over three times a day beats me. Some people say that you should eat 6–8 small meals a day. The problem with this is that when you fast in the evening, i.e., between dinner and breakfast, your body tries to burn fat that it has stored. We start the day off with a small meal, which releases insulin and stops fat from being broken down. The liver then starts storing glycogen; unfortunately, the liver has limited storage capacity and as a result, any excess glucose gets stored as fat (typically around your waistline). We eat one more meal, which pumps more glycogen into the liver before the glycogen in the liver from the previous meal runs out. When we eat over three meals a day, we don't give our bodies enough time to burn fat. We keep raising insulin levels in the blood, which causes fat to be stored and fat burning to stop. This is a surefire way to gain weight. The liver and pancreas are always going full speed, and they never get a break. How and when does the body use fat that has been stored? Answer– never.

At first glance, when you look at what insulin does, you might think that insulin is the main reason people gain weight. Not only does it stop your body from burning fat, but it also makes you make more fat, just think about it before you say anything, if Insulin always makes you gain weight, then why did we have such complicated processes? A complex set of hormones and enzymes, including insulin, work together to control how your body responds to food. For example, insulin stops the body from burning fat, while other hormones like glucagon, growth hormone, cortisol, and epinephrine make the body burn fat. And while insulin makes the body store fat, other hormones, like leptin, stop the body from storing fat. What we have at our hand is a complex interplay of hormones. We should not look at insulin in isolation.

Insulin isn't to blame. That's a short-sighted way to look at things. Insulin is important for regulating fat and glucose in a healthy person, like your grandfather, who lived to be 90 years old. Like other hormones, insulin is essential for the body to work well. insulin is a gift. Then comes the question of why insulin is a curse? The answer - When your body stops responding to insulin, i.e., insulin resistance.

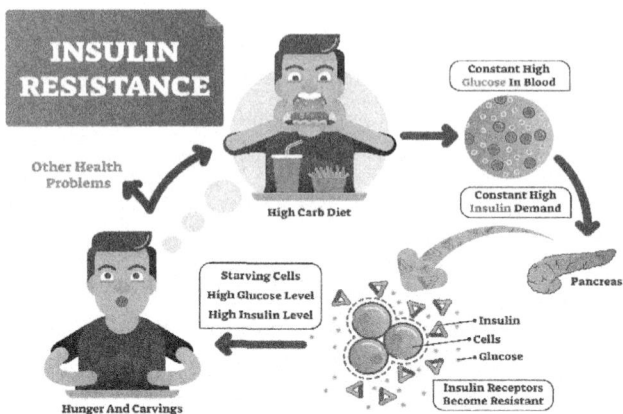

INSULIN RESISTANCE

Other Health Problems

High Carb Diet

Constant High Glucose In Blood

Constant High Insulin Demand

Pancreas

Starving Cells
High Glucose Level
High Insulin Level

Insulin
Cells
Glucose

Insulin Receptors Become Resistant

Hunger And Carvings

Insulin resistance is one of the main reasons people gain weight repeatedly. When our cells, liver, and other parts of our bodies don't respond well to insulin, we become resistant to it. insulin acts as a messenger. It tells cells to turn glucose into energy by sending messages to them. When cells can't respond to these messages, the pancreas has no choice but to make more insulin (i.e., more messages) in response to more glucose in the bloodstream.

Because of many factors and lifestyle over a long period, the pancreas has been constantly pumping insulin into the bloodstream, and for a long time, insulin levels have been high. When there is too much insulin, the cells get used to it and become less sensitive. Over time, they become resistant. Eventually, we get to a point where one insulin messenger isn't enough for a single cell. Instead, we need multiple insulin messengers for a single cell to release energy, and our insulin and glucose levels go up. The reason glucose levels are high is that the cell needs energy and isn't responding properly to the messenger (insulin). Cells that don't have enough energy look for more glucose, so we eat more to make up for the glucose shortage we think we have. This leads to more glucose in the bloodstream. The body will have to raise the amount of glucose in the bloodstream to meet the needs of the cells. Now, the pancreas senses that there is too much glucose in the blood and makes more insulin. This starts a vicious cycle that leads to high insulin and blood sugar perennially.

This raises the question of what happened first: did cells become less sensitive to insulin first, or did insulin levels rise first? Insulin resistance doesn't happen overnight; it can take years or even decades to show up. I talked about the sweet spot and how the body slowly changes it, as well as how weight goes up. (We shouldn't get too excited about the sweet spot theory, but it is a good way to understand how the body works). The body has some control, though, and this is based on the person's genes.

Insulin resistance is caused by both genetic and environmental factors, such as a diet high in simple carbohydrates, high levels of mental stress, not getting enough sleep, being inactive, etc. WHO[17] says that there are two main reasons for obesity: eating more high-calorie, high-sugar, and high-fat foods and not moving around enough. We also know that the liver can only store a certain amount of glycogen. Now, the liver works too hard and stores fat around the organs and around the waist. With insulin resistance, insulin makes the liver make more glycogen and fat, which makes the liver fat (i.e., fatty lever).

Our ancestors were healthy, people mostly used to die from things like wars, famine, not having enough health care, etc., and there were fewer obese people even 50 years ago. The Question is what has changed in the last 50 to 100 years? according to the WHO[18], since 1975, the number of obese people in the world have tripled.

Our ancestors knew how to deal with things like the type of food we eat, how often we eat, the effect of environmental stressors, not getting enough sleep, etc., but we don't seem to do the same. This is may be where we've gone wrong as a species. The key is to figure out what our ancestors did right and do the same things in our own lives.

Now that we know possible reason, let's fix it. In the following chapters, we'll try to figure out what might have caused the current situation and how to deal with it practically.

You may very well agree, we should take a long-term, all-around approach that is flexible and will last.

The suggested approaches should help, even for people who are predisposed to gain weight. The results may differ for each person, but with these methods, there will be a positive effect on the body and mind. You will definitely see results in a month or two, and the changes to your lifestyle are simple enough that you won't feel mentally drained. The best part is that this isn't a rule book, so you don't have to feel bad if you cheat or miss. Life is a great equalizer, in the long run, we will definitely have hits and misses, but we should celebrate the hits and learn from the misses. Once you really understand the ideas, it will be a lot easier to deal with difficult situations.

Chapter 4

Food: The Devil is in the details!

Chapter 4 - Food: The Devil is in the details!

The first step to living a healthy life is to know what we eat. Food is one thing we take for granted in life. The twenty-first century has given us a lot of food, and we live in a time when we can easily get food from all over the world.

If we want to live a healthy life, we need to know what we eat and how it affects our bodies. I mean, what's so great about knowing a few recipes for losing weight when you don't even know the "what" and "why" of the ingredients? You already know about carbs, proteins, and fat, you may also know that sugar is bad for you, etc., but have you ever tried to understand? Would you believe me if I said that carbs are not bad? If I told you that fat is good for your health and that everything you've heard about low-fat diets is wrong and not backed by science, would you believe me? Stay with me and be patient, and by the end of this chapter, I'm sure you'll know a few things that will make you proud.

What do we eat?

The food you eat can be put into two groups: macro and micro. Macro comprises carbs, protein, and fat. Micro being, minerals, and vitamins. Please keep in mind that this is a very simple way of looking at things, but I think this is enough to get the point across.

Macro Nutrients:

1. Carbohydrate:

As we already talked about (myth 1), carbs have a poor reputation among some dieters. Many people have gone as far as figuring out the exact amount of carbs that should be on a person's diet, and few supporters recommend cutting out all carbs. In the past few decades, there have been a lot of low-carb diets that have come and gone. I can easily think of the Ketogenic diet, the Atkins diet, the Low-carb-High-fat diet (LCHF), the Low-carb Paleo diet, the Zero-carb diet, and more.

It would take an entire book to talk about all the different carbohydrates. In the next few paragraphs, we'll inspect a few of the foods we eat every day and see how they affect us.

The name tells you what it's made of, doesn't it? Carbohydrate comes from the words "carbon" (carb) and "hydrate" (meaning a combination of hydrogen and oxygen).

Sugar, starch, and fiber are the three main types of

carbohydrates. Many authors divide carbs into simple and complex carbs, high-quality and low-quality carbs, or good and bad carbs. For ease of understanding, I would stick with the simple and complex carb analogy. Carbohydrates are grouped by how simple or complicated the carbon-hydrogen-oxygen chain is.

Carbohydrates with a single or double chain are called simple carbohydrates, i.e., monosaccharide or disaccharide (mono means one and saccharides means sugar and disaccharide means two sugar). Carbohydrates with over two chains are called polysaccharides, which means many sugars.

As a general rule, simple carbs are easy to break down and turn into glucose in the bloodstream. More chains of sugar make the carbohydrate hard to digest. The longer the chain, the more complex the carbohydrate. This makes it take longer for the body to break it down into glucose, which makes insulin release and the eases strain on the liver.

Simple carbs, also called single-dual chain carbs, are fructose (found in fruits) and galactose (found in milk), sucrose (table sugar), and maltose (found in beer and some vegetables). The glycemic index (or GI) is One of the best ways to figure out how much sugar is released in the blood. On a scale from 1 to 100, carbs with a GI of 100 are broken down the fastest, while carbs with a GI of 1 are broken down the slowest. Now, you might be interested in the GI of different sugars. The table below gives you an overview.

Sugar	GI value (approximate)
Glucose	100
Table sugar	65
Fructose	25
Lactose	40

Before you grab a bottle of fruit juice, i.e., Fructose, let's take each of these sugars apart to learn more about them.

Glucose:

We now know that the body's primary source of energy is glucose, and that every cell in the body needs glucose to work. The food we eat is turned into glucose by the body, which is then used as energy.

Sugar (white sugar, brown sugar, jaggery, etc.):

Sugar is a disaccharide, so it has two sugar molecules in it, one each of glucose and fructose. We'll talk about how fructose is broken down later. But because sugar is mostly glucose, it quickly raises the amount of glucose in the blood.

Table sugar, which is also called sucrose, comes from

the sugarcane plant and has become an essential part of our daily lives. Sugar seems to take up more space on the planet than any other substance. After cereals and rice, sugarcane is the third most valuable crop in the world. They grow it on 27 million hectares of land around the world. Aside from its economic wealth, the main thing it gives the world is a public health disaster that has been getting worse for hundreds of years. Obesity and diseases like cancer, dementia, heart disease, and diabetes that are linked to it and has spread to every country where sugar-based food has been the primary food source. So, it's important to look back and find out where sugar came from to understand how it became such a big problem.

The human body grew on a diet that was low in sugar and refined carbs. Sugar got into our food without us wanting it to. Most likely, Sugarcane was used to feed (or "fodder") for pigs. Why? To make the pig's fat! Sometimes, people ate the stalks recreationally. Evidence from plant remains and DNA shows that sugarcane came from Southeast Asia.

Around 3,500 years ago, sailors from Austronesia and Polynesia took the crop with them as they sailed across the Eastern Pacific and Indian Ocean. About 2,500 years ago, the first sugar that had been cleaned with chemicals was made in India. The method then moved east to China, then west to Persia, the first Islamic kingdoms and eventually to Europe.

Sugar is everywhere and makes up about 20% of the calories in our diets. It is also important to the global economy and cultural heritage.

Brazil makes the most sugar in the world, but India is the country that eats the most sugar. Brazil sends more than half of its crops abroad, but India produces and eats over 70% of its crops. [19]India is the world's capital of diabetes! India is also known as the world's capital of coronary heart disease. Both Diabetes and heart disease are linked to excessive sugar consumption.

Here are some of the bad things that table sugar does to our bodies (though research is still being done on this):

Weight - Increasing the amount of sugar you eat and drinking drinks with added sugars can cause you to gain weight. Research [20]has shown that adding sugar to our diets makes us more likely to have insulin resistance and coronary heart disease. If you eat a lot of foods that are high in sugar, you might gain weight faster. Studies have[21] shown that too much sugar can cause people to gain weight and become less sensitive to insulin. Another study [22]found that both children and adults who consume drinks with a lot of sugar gain weight and become obese.

Risk of eating too much: Foods with more sugar don't make you feel full because they lack fiber and other important nutrients. Glycemic load (GL) is important to understand. While glycemic index measures how quickly glucose gets into the bloodstream, glycemic load is a way to measure how many carbs you eat per serving. For example, 100 gms of watermelon has a high GI (72) and a low GL (3.6), while 100 grams of sugar has a high GI (65) and a high GL (75). This means that you would have to eat about 2 kg of watermelon to get the same amount of energy as sugar, in terms of calories, two teaspoons of sugar are the same as about 250 gms of watermelon. One can of Coca-Cola has about 40 gms of sugar, which is about the same as one KG of watermelon. Now consider the sugar you add to coffee/ tea every day. The worst part is that one KG of watermelon will keep you full for a long time, but this is not true of sugar. You get hungry quickly, and it's easy to overeat. Several short-term studies [23]have shown that solid carbohydrates are more filling than liquid carbohydrates; meaning it is easy to consume a bottle of sugary drink when compared with a loaf of bread.

Addictive: People all over the world love sugar. Several studies [24]have shown that sugar turns on parts of our brain that are linked to addiction and reward systems. This makes us want to eat sugary or high-energy foods. This mechanism worked well for hunters and gatherers, but it doesn't work well for modern people who have access to cheap sugar in large quantities.

Heart: People who eat or drink a lot of things with

sugar are more likely to get heart disease. Alarmingly, adding sugar is linked to a rise[25] in body fat and cholesterol levels in children, which makes them more likely to get heart problems.

Diabetes: Research shows that People who eat or drink a lot of sugary foods or drinks are more likely to get type 2 diabetes.

Tooth decay is more likely when you eat sugar, and high-sugar diets cause more tooth decay.

Bad breath: Too much sugar causes an imbalance in the oral microbiome, which comprises bacteria, which leads to bad breath.

Mood: Too many simple carbs can make you feel foggy-headed, depressed, anxious, and make it hard for you to think and remember things.

PCOS: Many studies have shown that higher insulin levels can cause an increase in androgen, which can lead to facial hair and acne and weight gain.

How can we get out of this? Is there no way out? The Problem is that you can't get rid of sugar in the world as it is now. The sugar content in biscuits, cookies, cereals, sweet treats, bread, bakery items, jams and ketchup, juices (even so-called fruit juices) and carbonated drinks, yoghurts (yes, read the label), ready-to-eat food and meal kits, etc., is between 15% and 75%. On average, and from what I've seen, almost all packaged food in the grocery store has sugar, even including the ones that say "digestive" or "fiber" or something similar.

Think about this: the average person eats between 150 and 350 gms of simple carbohydrates every day. This may not seem like much, but if you do the math for an entire year, you'll find that we eat between 50 to 90 kgs of simple carbs.

Even though it's hard to give up sugar, you can always control or limit how much you eat. It starts with small steps like cutting back on (or getting rid of) sugary snacks and drinks. Here are some things you can do to get rid of sugar:

How much sugar do you put in your tea or coffee? Start by cutting the amount of sugar you put in your tea or coffee to half and reduce the frequency. Strangely, coffee tastes best when there is no sugar in it. Have you tried it? You can also start by cutting the size of each serving (half glass instead of full glass). Try having a "no sugar day" once a week.

Practice mindful shopping at the supermarket. I have to say that I am also guilty of mindless shopping. Processed foods that are high in sugar are easy to find and cost little. When we look at a box of cookies, our minds do a quick calculation to tempt us to buy them. One clever way to shop mindfully is to prepare a list before entering the supermarket and try to stick with it as much as possible. Before putting anything in the basket, look at the labels and wait for 20 seconds.

Eliminate fruit juice and fizzy drinks. Yes, this is the change that is the easiest to make. They are unnecessary, they have a lot of sugar. A 600 ml bottle or can of coke has 65 gms of sugar. You don't think that's a lot, and you think I'm overreacting. Well, think about this: a teaspoon of sugar has 4-5 gms of sugar, so a can of Coke has 13–15 spoons of sugar. Would you add 15 teaspoons of sugar to your coffee? The American heart association says that men should have 9 teaspoons of sugar and women should have 6 teaspoons. Do you know why the heart association is telling people to eat less sugar? You know that the liver turns the sugar we eat into fats, which get into the bloodstream and lead to clogged arteries and result in heart ailments. In the next section, I'll talk about the so-called pure fruit juices. But the fruit juices you can buy at most grocery stores have a lot of added sugar. Pick up a bottle of mineral water instead of a fruit juice, there is no better way to quench your thirst than with natural water.

Be careful when you buy packaged foods that claim low sugar or no sugar. For example, a "sugar-free" cookie will still taste sweet if you try it. How? It has sugar substitutes that do more harm than good. Sugar free cookies have other hidden simple carbs such as ultra-processed flour that are same as sugar. Limit the amount of sweets and candy you eat during the day and only eat them when there's a special occasion.

An average person eats anywhere from 150 to 350 gms of simple carbs every day. This includes bread that says its whole wheat, but wheat only makes up 15–50% of the total weight. This may not seem like much, but if you do the math for an entire year, you'll find that we eat between 50 and 90 kgs of simple carbs.

Some of you might be angry that I put the jaggery along with sugar. Since the beginning of time, they have taught us that jaggery is naturally full of trace minerals and is good for the body. However, in terms of glycemic index and load, Jaggery is same as sugar. For example:

There is a difference between eating real oranges and drinking orange juice (more on this in the next chapter).

Like table sugar, jaggery puts the same amount of stress on the bloodstream and insulin.

Jaggery may only have a psychological advantage when compared with table sugar and makes no difference from an insulin load perspective.

Fructose:

Fructose is a natural sugar that can be found in fruit, honey, high fructose corn syrup, agave nectar, maple syrup, and other similar sources. In the last 100 years, fructose consumption and production have increased by many times. It has 73% more sweetness than sugar. Fructose is also called fruit sugar and is found in many fruits' plants, flowers, root vegetables, nectar, and sugar cane

Researchers[26] found that fructose is digested, absorbed, and used in the same way as glucose and table sugar. Fructose has a very low GI, which means it doesn't turn into glucose in the bloodstream and doesn't make insulin levels go up. Also, fructose is sweeter than sugar, so people can use less of it per serving. Fructose was and still is a great alternative to table sugar, which led to the growth of a booming industry based on lies. Fructose got more attention with the development of High Fructose Corn Syrup (HFCS) as a liquid alternative to sugar where it was synthesized and extracted from corn. Most of the added sugar in processed foods (such as soda drinks and processed foods) comes from HFCS. 42% to 55% of HCFS is fructose, and the other half is glucose. Honey is 54% fructose and 46% glucose, while table sugar is 50% glucose and 50% fructose. But, Agave syrup is different because 75% of it is fructose and the other 25% is glucose. However, the Agave syrup you can buy in stores only has 56% fructose, you should instead look for pure or unprocessed agave syrup. So, there is no difference at all between regular table sugar, agave syrup, and the HCFS that is added to processed foods.

On the one hand, the intestine breaks down glucose, which then gets into the bloodstream and is taken up by the cells. The liver breaks down fructose, which is then taken to the cells. The only good thing about fructose is that it doesn't cause insulin to be released like glucose does.

A question will arise: what is the harm in consuming fructose? Such as a few glasses of orange juice or homemade fruit juice. The European Food Safety Authority [27]said that fructose may be better than sucrose and glucose in sugar-sweetened foods and drinks because it has less of an effect on postprandial blood sugar levels. However, they also said that "high intakes of fructose may lead to metabolic complications such as dyslipidemia, insulin resistance, and type 2 diabetes." The advice clarifies that eating a moderate amount of fructose as part of a healthy diet is fine, but it does not recommend eating a lot of fructose.

What happens when we eat too much fructose? When a person eats too much fructose, the liver can't process it quickly. Instead, it turns fructose into fat (de novo lipogenesis), which [28] is carried through the bloodstream and stored as fat. Studies have shown that eating too much fructose can make you hungrier because it makes it harder for your body to use insulin and blocks the hormone that makes you feel hungry. The liver will also have to work harder, which can lead to a rare condition called fatty liver, which is usually seen in alcoholics.

If fructose is bad, what about fruits? There is a difference between eating fruit and just drinking fruit juice, even if the juice is pure or cold-pressed.

When sugar is mixed with its natural fiber, like in a whole fruit, it takes longer to digest, and up to 30% of the fructose does not get absorbed in the small intestine. Instead, the fructose is broken down by microorganisms in the large intestine, improving overall microbial diversity and help prevent disease. The fiber will also make the blood sugar rises more slowly.

Take orange juice as an example. Let's say it has no added sugar and is in its natural state (i.e., pure juice). Orange juice has fructose, and as we've already said, it takes about 5–6 oranges to make concentrated juice, one glass of orange juice is easy to drink all at once, but can you eat 5 or 6 oranges at once? No, you don't. You get full sooner rather than later. Fiber is the secret ingredient because it makes you feel full. Compared to drinking one glass of orange juice, it's less likely that you'll eat six oranges all at once. Even though juice can make you feel full quickly, it has a downside: it's easy to drink too much of it, and your body won't have to work hard to turn it into fat, so you'll be hungry again soon. The best thing to drink instead of fruit juice is a smoothie with no added sugar because it has the whole fruit, not just the juice.

Lactose:

Lactose is a sugar found in dairy milk. It is a disaccharide, meaning it has two sugar molecules namely, Glucose and Galactose. It is broken down and synthesized in the intestine and absorbed into the bloodstream.

Lactose is in the milk that we drink. Milk has the lowest GI of any food, at 40, and it breaks down slowly. It also helps the body absorb vitamins and minerals better. Dairy and lactose are not known to elicit alarming insulin response in humans and should be safe to consume in moderation.

Ultra-processed food:

What do roti, naan, bread, rolls, crackers, cookies, tortillas, cakes, pastries, muffins, donuts, noodles and pasta, and white rice all have in common? These fall into a unique category of ultra-processed foods (UPF). This is an in-between carbohydrate that people have made by removing all the naturally occurring fiber, vitamins, and minerals from the carbohydrate, like in white flour or white rice.

UPF is very similar to sugar in the it acts, absorbed, and insulin release.

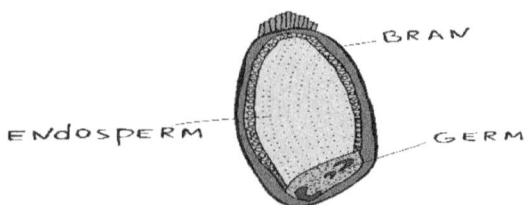

BRAN
ENDOSPERM
GERM

For example, A grain of wheat has three parts: the bran, which is mostly fiber and the wheat's outer covering; the germ, which is the embryo of the seed and is high in protein and nutrients; and the endosperm, which is mostly starch, has the most carbohydrate and the least amount of nutrients. In the modern milling process, the bran, embryo, and most of the nutrients are taken out of the wheat while the endosperm is kept, the endosperm is then bleached with chemicals, which makes the flour white. So, what's left is a powder that is high in simple carbohydrate but low in nutrients. The result is that the intestine absorbs carbohydrates quickly, which causes a rise in blood sugar and, along with it, insulin. Fact is, our ancestors did not have access to modern-day milling, all they had was grinding stones where stripping was not possible, and the grains were coarsely grounded and not finely powdered. Why do you think medicines, both old and new, come in fine powder form? The reason is that the contact area of the medicine with the body is increased, resulting in faster absorption and higher bioavailability. In the same way, when flour is ground up into a fine powder, it is absorbed more quickly, which causes blood glucose levels to rise quickly.

When I was a child, flour was ground at home or at a stone mill. I also remember my grandmother insisting that the flour be ground coarsely. When I asked her why she wanted the flour course, she would say "to help digestion", when I asked how does it help digestion, she did not have an answer she. After a lot of questioning, she finally said that this was how her mother did it. She had the knowledge passed from many generations that grinding flour coarsely results in slowing down digestion and delays glucose release.

Bottom line:

Sugar is naturally occurring or artificially synthesized. Eating too much refined sugar and UPF is bad for you and may have a negative effect in the long run. Modern industries make sure that UPF doesn't have any minerals, fiber, or other naturally occurring substances in it. This makes it easy to taste and absorb, which causes a rise in blood sugar and an insulin response. This is especially bad for people who already have a condition like insulin resistance, obesity, being overweight, a heart condition, diabetes, etc., because our bodies turn sugar into fat easily and quickly. Simple carbs are a big reason people gain weight and have a higher chance of getting heart disease and type 2 diabetes.

Even though it sounds hard, we can control and cut back on sugar and UPF by making simple, easy-to-do changes in our lives. Yes, it's hard to give up sugar and UPF; although it is okay to treat yourself once in a while, we get into trouble when we make a lifestyle out of UPF and sugar.

The key is to eat as little sugar and UPF as possible. I am reminded of the verse in the Bhagavad Gita I alluded to in the foreword. Unfortunately, ancient humans (Bhagwad Gita dates back to 3000 BC) did not have access to sugar and UPF! Given today's situation, we could rephrase the verse and say that we should consume processed food frugally and rest of the food moderately!

I know it's easier to say something than to do it. We've tried many times and failed. Trying to stop is especially hard when there is a lot of sugar or UPF around. We can't get sugar or UPF to zero, but the question is how much we can cut back? We might stay away from sugar or UPF for a few days or a month, but all it takes is one stressful event or an uncontrollable craving, and the whirlpool will swallow us up in the blink of an eye.

Well, here are a few things that will happen if you could control sugar/UPF.

Sugar and UPF make you hungry, and limiting the amount of sugar you eat will help stabilize your blood sugar and make insulin resistance easier to deal with.

To refresh, insulin resistance makes you crave for more sugar. Control sugar and insulin stabilizes.

You will start losing weight within a few weeks because you have lost water and fat. Yes, your waistline will reduce!

Have you ever felt tired after a meal? Sugar is to blame. Cut back on sugar, and you'll feel less tired and more awake after a meal.

Sugar and hormones are linked directly. As having more insulin affects the amount of testosterone in men and estrogen in women. As soon as you cut down on sugar, your skin will look better (for females as androgens increase acnes and reduction in androgens will cause better skin condition).

From the point of view of how your body burns fat, there will be a tectonic shift, and changes will happen at the level of the cells.

You are cleansing your liver; remember, your liver is on an overdrive and accumulating fat in and around it. By cutting down sugar, you will give your liver a breather.

Will power gets too much credit. We don't seem to have control over our minds; instead, our minds have more power over us. So, what should we do? Are we struck? The more we try to stop wanting something, the more our mind wants it. It's hard to break the sugar/UPF habit. There are no rules from the governments on sugar and UPF other than difficult to read labeling. The common man does not perceive any threat to sugar/ UPF. Although we are fully aware of its dangers[29], all it takes is the smell of a freshly baked cookie and our minds trick us into eating a lot of them. It's not all bad news! In the "mind over body" chapter, I'll give you a few tips you can use right away.

Off topic a bit, Rice has always interested me. All the important nutrients and fiber are taken out of polished or white rice, which makes it a UPF. However, Rice is one of the most popular grains in the world, and Asians eat almost 90% of the world's rice crop. Nearly three billion people around the world eat rice every day. Almost all the rice that is consumed is processed, i.e., white rice. Before the western diet, most rice-eating countries had much lower rates of obesity than they do now. For example, China makes and eats the most rice, but it ranks 191st in terms of obesity, and Bangladesh, which eats the most rice per person, ranks 195th. Most of the recent rise in obesity in China is because western diet encroachment.

I have seen rice being eaten in many countries, and it is definitely more than the recommended levels. People are not overweight. Does that mean it's safe to eat white rice? Question is, how? There is no simple answer to this question, but the following could be probable reasons:

As we've already talked about, the western fast-food diet is full of highly processed foods and has a shocking amount of sugar and salt. But a normal household in Asia is not likely to have the same amount of sugar/ UPF.

Some people can break down rice well, while others can do it better with wheat.

In terms of obesity, the east is behind the west because most people in west are already overweight. In the east, people are still catching up.

Along with rice, the Asian diet includes a healthy amount of greens, vegetables, pulses, whole grains and healthy meat. Except rice, the rest of the diet is unprocessed. Also, the spices that are used as part of Asian Cuisine may slow down digestion (cardamom, cinnamon and other spices have proven slow digestion properties). Even though there is rice in the diet, that doesn't make it less healthy. If you don't believe me, you can see for yourself at any Asian restaurant.

When knowledge is passed down from generation to generation, the food made at home is balanced and healthy. Also, an average Asian diet doesn't have any sugar in it every day. Sugar is something they eat occasionally, but not every day. They save sweet treats for holidays and other special events.

How do greens and vegetables help compensate? The

answer is complex carbs.

Complex carbs:

Before we can figure out what complex carbs are, we need to learn about the gut microbiome, which comprises the bacteria and other micro-organisms that live in your gut. The term "microbiome" refers to the trillions of bacteria, archaea, viruses, fungi and protozoa, collectively known as the gut microbiota that live on and inside us and. Around 100 trillion microbes live in our guts (hence the name gut microbiome or microbiota. A person weighing 70 kg (155 pounds) has about 1-2 kg of microbiota in their colon. The human genome has about 23,000 genes, while the gut microbiota has about 3 million genes all together[30]. So, in terms of genes, microbiota outnumbers us. As humans have developed and changed what they eat, so have the microbiota, and it will continue to change and grow. From birth until death, the gut microbiome and humans have worked well together. They function like an organ in the body. They help you digest food, affect your weight, control your behavior, lower or raise your anxiety (the gut is called the second brain), make neurotransmitters that travel through your bloodstream to your brain and change how your brain works, and keep your immune system in check. Scientists have found that the brain and the gut can talk back and forth with each other. For example, people who are too stressed out may get an upset stomach, and the microbiota in the gut may affect mood, motivation, and even cognitive function, such as decision making. Several studies have shown that microbiota affects personality traits and social behavior. The link is complicated, and research is still growing and in its early stages, but the connection is clear. There are a lot of good and bad microbes in the microbiota[31]. Studies [32]have shown that making bad choices about what to eat and lifestyle can throw the balance between good and bad microbes off, which can lead to weight gain.

We have all, without a doubt, experienced the nexus at some point or another. Based on what a person eats, the microbiota can change quickly, and a few species may go extinct or new species can come into existence. Losing a few species may not seem like a big deal, but in the medium to long term, any change in the microbiota's diversity could cause metabolic diseases, inflammatory bowel syndrome, psychiatric disorders like depression and anxiety, and other health problems. The intestinal microbiota can influence our metabolism. Lifestyle changes such as going on a diet, taking antibiotics disturbs microbiota composition, and hence the metabolic activity of the microbiota can affect our body mass by either boosting weight gain or help in losing weight. For example, research [33]has shown that the use of antibiotics in early life leads to obesity. Why am I talking about this? Think back to the chapter on diet and think about how diet might affect the microbiota. Well, think about this: more and more research [34]suggests that one of the major causes of obesity is the loss of biodiversity.

Pasteurization (more on this in the fermentation chapter), the use of antibiotics, and ultra-processed ready-to-eat food have all had a big effect on the microbiota, where we have changed the ecosystem to our detriment in the last century.

The microbiota in your gut can stay healthy if you eat a lot of fiber and resistant starch or complex carbs. Researchers[35] have found that the microbiota in our guts love fibers and complex carbs. For example, they form a protective mucosal layer that protects the colon lining.

What are complex carbs? Let's figure it out in the next few paragraphs.

Starch and fiber are two examples of Complex carbs. Let's start with starch, which is the most important and most underrated carbohydrate. Dieticians write little about starch, and most people think it's just as bad as sugar. Still, 60% to 70% of all calories in the world come from starch.

Starch is a polysaccharide, where "poly" means "many" and "saccharide" means "sugar." Starch comprises many strands of glucose. Plants make starch to store energy. Plants store this extra energy in different ways, such as tubers in potatoes and sweet potatoes, tapioca (sago pearls are made from tapioca), seeds of corn, rice, wheat, millets, oats, barley, all kinds of beans, and dicot seeds, lentils, peas, chickpeas, etc. Many fossils studies have shown that our hunter-gatherer ancestors ate mostly uncooked and unprocessed starches. Starch has always been an important source of energy for humans, and it still is. The intestine turns starch into glucose, which is used for energy. Strangely, not all starch is quickly broken down and turned into glucose. Starch can be put into three major groups: rapidly digestible (RDS), slowly digestible (SDS), and resistant (RS).[36].

I would like to elaborate RS though as RDS and SDS are self-explanatory.

Pulses (beans, peas, black gram, green gram, groundnut, lentils, and so on) deserve special attention.

One of the simplest ways to remember pulses is that their seeds normally split into two equal halves (hence the name dicots). There are a few exceptions, such as cashew and almond, which are not pulses.

Whole pulses are high in protein, complex carbohydrate (starch), and fiber (more on fiber in the next chapter).

In India, a country divided between rice and wheat, there is widespread consumption of pulses, with pulses being part of both vegetarian and non-vegetarian daily diets. Pulses are India's proxy staple. Beans and peas are consumed daily around the world. Global pulse production and consumption are both increasing. Starch accounts for over 80% of the carbohydrates found in pulses.

One question that demands an answer is, contrary to common assumption, how is starch a staple for such a vast population if it is responsible for obesity and weight gain? The answer is resistant starch (RS), and pulses are high in RS.

RS does not get metabolized in the small intestine and instead goes to the large intestine, where it is broken down by bacteria.

In the small intestine, RS transforms into a thin mucous fluid before passing to the large intestine. The microbiota in the large intestine ferment or eat the starch, which makes fatty acids that the microbiota uses as their source of energy and the fatty acids are also absorbed by the colon cells.

The impact is essentially twofold: RS does not raise blood glucose levels since it [37]has a low glycemic index, lowering insulin production, and RS enhances satiety due to its ability to absorb water and tendency to form mucus, resulting in less overeating and snacking.

Pulses are the finest source of RS because they contain more than half of the starch. Cooking pulses diminishes RS to some level since RS is degraded during cooking; cooling pulses to room temperature restores RS to a great extent.

Even if you ingest pulses hot, there is still plenty of RS (although partially destroyed) from which you could derive benefit.

For thousands of years, Indians have fermented and consumed pulses, and the expertise got passed down from generation to generation.

Fermentation offers several advantages, including boosting the nutritious content of the pulses, improving color, flavor, texture, and palatability, and increasing protein availability. In a subsequent chapter, we shall learn more about fermentation.

Here are a few benefits of RS:

1. Researchers 38have found that they can help keep the health of the colon in good shape.
2. Components of small chain fatty acids not absorbed by cells of colon are used by the small intestine and liver for metabolism
3. Prevents colon cancer.
4. Playing a key role in cross-talk between the gut and the brain.
5. Insulin sensitivity (39 and 40)is improved. Insulin sensitivity is the opposite of insulin resistance, meaning, the cells are receptive to insulin vis-à-vis

resistive in case of insulin resistance (although not extensively researched, it may eventually help in weight loss).

6. Increasing the feeling of fullness, cutting down on the amount of food eaten, and delaying the next meal.

Here are some starches that come from nature:

1. RS is found in grains, beans, seeds, and other foods.
2. RS is found in potato, unripe banana, sweet potato, yam, etc.
3. Resistant starch is formed when certain starchy foods are cooked and chilled, such as cooked and cooled potato and rice, also referred to as retrogradation41.
4. It has also been observed 42that certain cooking methods, including43 steaming, boiling, microwave heating, and frying, can promote resistant starch, but pressure cooking has an opposite effect.

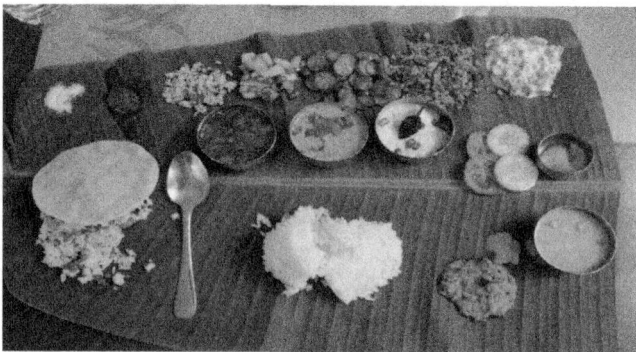

In the southern part of India, we can see a balanced

diet and the importance of pulses in any traditional house during a special event or festival. Most of the time, food is served on a plantain leaf where food is arranged from left to right and top to bottom. On the top left are two cooked salads and two raw salads. Pulses and cucumber are the most important parts of the raw salad. People are supposed to eat the raw salad first. Also, there are boiled lentils at the right bottom, which should be eaten with rice at the start of the meal. The ingredients and the order in which you eat them may have been chosen to balance carbohydrate, fullness, and nutrition. We have done this for many years without realising how important it is. The way food is set out and how it is eaten is so well thought out that it balances the diet, the calories, and the nutrition. This is just an illustration, there are similar examples all over India and the world, across all cultures, of how our ancestors ate in a way that was perfectly balanced for their environment, the seasons, their culture, and their body types. This means that you already had a customized diet, and it's a shame that we now have to look in books for the perfect diet. Since the beginning of time, they taught us how to live healthily. We just forgot about it.

People of all cultures around the world eat raw fruits like bananas, mangoes, jackfruits, etc. Do you know what the benefits are?

The amount of RS and fiber in a Raw or green banana

is high. The acids in the stomach and enzymes in the small intestine can 't break the starch[44]. The Banana Stem is eaten in many places. The stem has 40–50% starch and is about 15% RS[45].

In many tropical and subtropical countries around the world, [46]Raw jackfruit is a common food. Jackfruit seeds are also a common food in many native cultures. Raw jackfruit and its seeds contain large amount of RS.

In the same way, many cultures around the world eat unripe mango, durian, breadfruit, etc. as part of their diet. I haven't done a thorough analysis of the research in this area, but these foods may also have high RS.

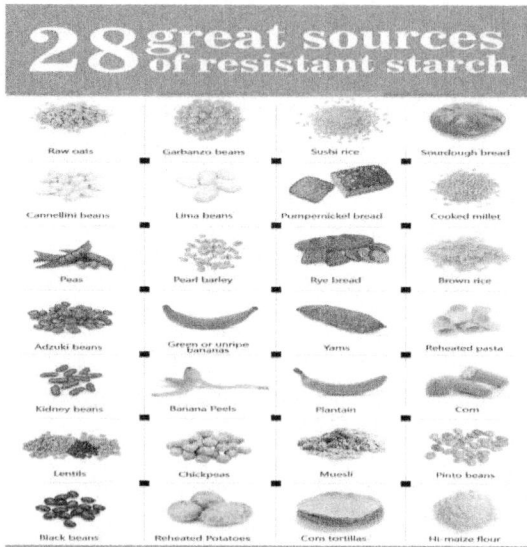

28 great sources of resistant starch

Raw oats	Garbanzo beans	Sushi rice	Sourdough bread
Cannellini beans	Lima beans	Pumpernickel bread	Cooked millet
Peas	Pearl barley	Rye bread	Brown rice
Adzuki beans	Green or unripe bananas	Yams	Reheated pasta
Kidney beans	Banana Peels	Plantain	Corn
Lentils	Chickpeas	Muesli	Pinto beans
Black beans	Reheated Potatoes	Corn tortillas	Hi maize flour

Are you still not sure? Here are a few more advantages:

1. RS helps prevent[47] colon cancer, stops fat from building up, may help prevent gallstones, improves mineral absorption, and lowers blood sugar. These things have a direct effect on weight management.
2. RS can lower[48] cholesterol and triglyceride levels in the blood.

We'll end the chapter on carbohydrates with a look at fiber.

Fiber is a carbohydrate that our bodies cannot digest. It behaves similarly to starch, in that it cannot be broken down into sugars. Fiber bypasses the digestive tract and ends up in the large intestine, where the microbiota ferments and brakes it down.

Fiber is water soluble (found in oatmeal, nuts, beans, apples, and blueberries) or insoluble (found on the skins of seeds, fruits, and vegetables), meaning it does not dissolve in water.

Soluble fiber, like RS, draws water in the stomach and creates a gel-like material, slowing digestion and increasing satiety.

Cholesterol is lowered by soluble fiber because it binds to it in the small intestine. Once the fiber gets to the small intestine, it sticks to the cholesterol particles and keeps them from getting into the bloodstream and going to other parts of the body ([49] and [50]).

Soluble fiber lowers cholesterol because the liver

utilizes cholesterol to generate bile acids. Soluble fiber binds to bile acids, limiting bile acid availability for the liver. The liver next shifts to the blood, where it draws cholesterol from the circulation for bile production, resulting in a decrease in free-flowing cholesterol in the blood. The symbiotic relationship with the gut microbiota and the beneficial effect of fiber are like that of RS.

As a side note, several people have asked me about the meat-based diet and how our ancestors survived without fiber, as well as whether we should have fiber at all? There are few societies or populations that have entirely relied on meat for their calorie requirements. Meat has always been an important part of the human diet for protein, micronutrients, and fat, but never for energy, as people (even heavy meat eaters) have always consumed carbs, and the carbohydrates that our forefathers ingested were never ultra-processed!

Bottom line: Carbohydrates are an important part of a healthy diet since they give energy, fiber, nutrition, and excellent source of starch. Removing or severely reducing carbohydrate (low carb and high-fat diet) from the diet is a self-defeating strategy because you are also removing the goodness of fiber, nutrients, and starch. Recommendation is to consume beans, lentils, whole grains, potatoes, sweet potatoes, and other nutrient-dense foods as part of a well-balanced diet.

Protein

The protein's makeup is carbon, hydrogen, oxygen, and nitrogen organised as amino acid strands. Amino acids are protein building components; the arrangement of the amino acids (carbon, hydrogen, oxygen, nitrogen, and sometimes sulphur) dictates the protein's structure and chemical properties.

There are around twenty amino acids, nine of which are deemed necessary for humans because the body cannot synthesize them on its own and must be supplemented by food.

Protein, contrary to popular perception, is not just used to build muscle. Proteins are required for a variety of bodily processes. The human body needs a certain amount of protein for tissue maintenance. Every cell in the human body uses protein, including muscles, bones, organs, tendons, ligaments, and so on. Protein is also needed for the production of enzymes, antibodies, hormones, blood-clotting cells, and for blood transport. The body is in perpetual change, with its tissues constantly being renewed and repaired where protein is essential for this activity.

The amount of protein consumed by an individual varies depending on a variety of parameters, such as exercise level, age, muscle mass, and so on, and is never consistent across humans.

Protein, as you may have seen, shares molecular similarities with carbs, and hence, protein can be used by the body to produce energy and fat (you read it right, the body can convert protein to fat). And the opposite is true as well where the body can convert protein to energy; typically occurring during starvation or calorie restricted diets.

Protein overconsumption can cause weight gain and fat deposition. Protein is a key macronutrient in terms of weight management; research suggests that when ingested in moderation, it can promote satiety and aid in weight management. However, [51]Protein is over-hyped and positioned as a miracle macronutrient for muscle building and weight management. Our forefathers used to receive protein through meat, fish, dairy, legumes, and so on; now we have protein bars, protein shakes, whey protein, soy protein, and array of similar processed supplements.

Protein synthesis and processing is a niche business in which entrepreneurs use creative technologies to artificially manufacture protein. Bodybuilding has been an obsession in recent decades, and men are looking for ultra-short cuts to build muscles.

I've seen gym attendees consume protein blindly, with little regard for the amount of workout they're doing or their body demand. Your doctor rarely recommends protein supplements because protein deficiency does not occur frequently.

Although policymakers frequently recommend daily

protein intake as part of a balanced diet, supplements are rarely recommended. Another issue with supplements is that they are not regulated, therefore neither your doctor nor the regulator may prescribe a dosage for supplemental protein. You're at the mercy of your personal trainer!

Unlike fat, our bodies are not built to store extra protein as muscle. Any additional protein will be turned into fat and increase your need for a bathroom break as frequent urination is side effect of excessive protein consumption. Unfortunately, fitness fanatics are innocent and are duped by an industry that purposely creates fake demand.

A protein bar is often two or three times the price of a regular bar, although the components used in the bar are typically soy protein, which is the cheapest type of protein and is typically used as an animal feed. Soy (together with palm oil) is the leading cause of deforestation and is farmed in the most unscientific and unethical ways possible.

Unassuming customers are being outwitted and tricked at their own game, while shareholders profit at the price of consumers' health. Protein bars, ironically, are far from healthy, and they harm your system more than anything else.

Because Protein bars are heavily processed, they are heavy in palm oil (or other vegetable oil), corn syrup, a slew of preservatives and antioxidants (toxic chemicals). Why should someone put those substances into their system is the question? Perhaps The answer is carbohydrate and fat paranoia.

Aside from the hazards mentioned above, here are a few other risks associated with supplementary protein consumption:

Because the Protein supplement market is unregulated, you are at the mercy of the manufacturers. What they claim may not be true, and even the tiny language on the labels reveals little.

A high-protein diet[52] may put a strain on the kidneys, reduce bone mass and density, and raise the risk of calcium accumulation in the urinary tract. Many animal protein supplements are high in saturated fat, which may be harmful to heart health.

There are no standard protein intake prescriptions. Protein intake dosages are frequently prescribed by non-health professionals such as your trainer who is unaware of how your body metabolises protein, your protein requirement, your proclivity to add muscle, protein intake as part of diet and the resultant deficit based on your workout regimen, and so on.

It impairs your digestive and metabolic functioning.

It has the potential to alter your gut microbiome, often resulting in irreparable damage.

What are our options?

Instead of bars, shakes, and powders, there are much healthier ways to get protein; meat, poultry, dairy, seeds, and vegetables, to name a few. It is also important to note that there is enough and more protein in a balanced diet and there is no need to consume supplements unless your health care professional recommends it.

Over the last few decades, there has been an inordinate emphasis on animal protein, resulting in spiraling meat consumption and a spiraling poultry business. Meat has contributed to deforestation and global warming.

Our forefathers gained their daily protein fix from a combination of meat, vegetables, and grains (not meat alone).

And, in many parts of the world (aside from a few malnourished people), there is a sizable vegan/vegetarian community whose daily protein intake is derived primarily from plants and dairy; there has never been a protein shortage for this population.

2. Fat

All macronutrients have one thing in common: they are combinations of carbon, hydrogen, and oxygen. Fat has the highest energy density per ounce of the three, which may explain why the body transforms and stores carbs as fat. We all know that human dietary fat is sourced from either plant (peanut oil, linseed oil, canola oil, olive oil, and so on) or animals (diary fats, animal fats, etc.,).

Saturated fat, unsaturated fat, and trans-fat are the three types of fat.

Saturated fats are generated from carbon molecules that establish a strong connection with hydrogen molecules, making them "saturated." Saturated fats are easy to remember since they are solid at room temperature (coconut oil, clarified butter etc.,). Unsaturated fat is one that lacks few hydrogen bonds. Trans-fat does not occur naturally and is manufactured. We discovered an amazing approach to chemically saturate unsaturated fat using a process called hydrogenation, which involves artificially saturating carbon with a hydrogen molecule.

Fats have had a poor rap and are thought to be unhealthy. Obesity, high cholesterol, and other health issues are blamed on fat consumption.

Even today, many governments, health care experts, dietitians, and doctors believe that eating fat above specific limits is unhealthy. We still have best-selling diet books that advocate a low-fat diet. When you go to the supermarket, you will notice low-fat yoghurt, low-fat chips/ crisps, low-fat cookies/ biscuits, and the list goes on. Packaged food labels should include a breakdown of saturated, trans, and unsaturated fat content.

As you will see in the following chapter, the human body is a fat producing factory, and it produces fat in excess in overweight persons. Even if you don't consume dietary fat, your body will produce fat. Even if you don't consume any oil, your liver manufactures cholesterol.

The question is why? Cholesterol, a fat-like waxy substance helps your body make certain essential substances such as cell membranes, hormones (including testosterone and estrogen), vitamin D, etc.

When someone has a lipid profile test, the result may show excessive cholesterol, but it will never show cholesterol from dietary food or liver; fact is, the liver primarily produced it. Perhaps the reason we have more cholesterol is not because we eat more fat, but because our liver produces fat at an alarming rate.

The reason our liver is producing excessive fat is because of excessive sugar and ultra-processed food in our diet. The culprit, therefore, is ultra-processed food and sugar, which our liver constantly converts to fat (or cholesterol). After all, it's not the fat we eat that's the problem!

If you still don't believe it, studies have proven that cholesterol levels in humans progressively grow with age, and increased cholesterol levels are not unusual in persons aged 65 to 75. Although cholesterol is a risk factor for those who are vulnerable, it becomes less of a concern after the age of 75. According to the study, there is evidence that high total cholesterol is connected with longevity. All of my relatives over the age of 65 have high cholesterol and are on statins.

I am not saying that we ignore cholesterol; rather, before deciding, one should always consult with a physician. My point here is that we should consider fat in a broader context, and blaming dietary fat alone for elevated cholesterol is inappropriate. Rather than focusing on fat, we should instead focus on a comprehensive diet and controlling sugar/UPF.

Government standards, product labels, and fragmented studies have confused rather than helped the public. Saturated fat, for example, is directly related to elevated cholesterol levels in the body. There is also evidence that suggests saturated fat may contribute to heart disease. Contradictory studies and outcomes add to the confusion.

For example, the American Heart Association suggests limiting saturated fats to 5% to 6% of daily calorie consumption; while I am sure much study has gone into this suggestion, it is unclear how 5% to 6% is measured daily. It's both impossible and unlikely. How can one focus on quantity daily? Despite these recommendations, the global prevalence of heart disease, obesity, type 2 diabetes, and linked disorders has increased. Does it mean that fat consumption has increased drastically? No - With all the focus on fat, we may have overlooked the unassuming culprit: "carbs" in processed foods, which are directly accountable and had a significant influence. Does this imply that we might follow a high-fat diet? No - Several studies have showed that a high-fat diet poses a considerable danger to overall health (albeit research is still in its early stages and more has to be done) such as:

1. Increased oxidative stress and mitochondrial malfunction in several tissues, causing organ stress.
2. Accelerates age-related hearing loss.
3. Inflammation of the small intestine.

Ironically, I am tempted to return to the Bhagawad Gita, saying that food should be consumed in moderation. You should think twice before embarking on a low or high-fat diet.

Micro Nutrients:

Micronutrients, as the name implies, are nutrients that are necessary for humans but are required in lesser amounts than macronutrients. The primary micronutrients are vitamins and minerals. Some vitamins are not produced by our bodies and must get from plants and animals. We get the vitamins and minerals that plants and animals make or take in when we eat them. Vitamins and minerals are essential for the proper functioning of the organism.

We all know that vitamins A, B, C, D, E, and so on, and that minerals such as calcium, phosphorus, potassium, sodium, chloride, magnesium, iron, zinc, iodine, sulphur, cobalt, copper, fluoride, manganese, and selenium are necessary.

Because there is no single technique to calculate the number of micronutrients in each item, it is critical to have a diverse and well-balanced diet. I won't go into depth on how important vitamins and minerals are and what happens when you don't get enough of them because you may already know some of this or be able to learn more about it.

In the following lines, I'd like to discuss how soil degradation promotes micronutrient loss in the fruits and vegetables we eat. Yes, meat eaters may have an upper hand over vegetarians and vegans since meat provides critical micronutrients. However, there are hazards to eating plain meat, which we will discuss later.

You go to the supermarket and buy an orange. It looks like an orange. When you eat it after peeling off the skin, it tastes like an orange and is quite sweet. But are you certain that the orange provides the same quantity of vitamins and minerals? The issue is that there isn't much information available on the nutritional value and density of the present-day foods.

Yes, you can find nutritional information about a fruit,

vegetable, or even meat on the internet, but no one knows when the analysis was performed, where the fruit or vegetable or meat comes from, what the soil is like, how it was grown, or if the meat came from wild, free-range, grass-fed, or grain-fed animals. There is no way to assess or determine how ethical the farmers were when growing the food.

Fruits and vegetables may have had substantially more nutrition and micronutrients even just a few ago compared to the diet we eat now. The only reason our food may contain fewer nutrients is because the land is depleted of nutrients.

Because of the large number of people who needed to be fed and the scarcity of food following World War II, certain governments were forced to employ contemporary intensive agriculture methods.

These approaches include, but are not limited to, using hybrid varieties of crops with more calories per gram of grain, making food more palatable, using chemical fertilisers, pesticides, insecticides, and herbicides, and encouraging monoculture over bio diversity.

Although the green revolution has resulted in a significant boost in output, allowing us to feed over 7 billion people and combat world hunger, it has come at a cost: soil loss and erosion.

The Green Revolution provided calories, but it may

not have provided nutrition. People may question what soil depletion and micronutrient loss have in common. Herbicides, insecticides, and pesticides applied to or near soil (i.e., on the plant) has degraded the soil.

Soil is rich in microbes and other forms of life (bacteria, fungus, earthworms, and so on) that coexists with plants. Microbes and fungi, for example, assist plants in obtaining nutrients in a usable form. This interaction permits the plant to absorb nutrients.

Plants are better able to break down the nutrients in the soil through their symbiotic relationship with the soil and its microbes, where they change the nutrients that are present in the soil and rock. Scientists have only scratched the surface of how plants and microorganisms interact. Soil is now nothing more than a place for plants to grow. Modern farming, for example, is causing soil degradation:

Using nitrogen, phosphorous, and phosphate fertilisers causes the soil to become acidic. Because pesticides are used on plants, pests are getting resistant to them. This has resulted in a never-ending war against pests, with pesticide companies developing stronger and more lethal chemicals. There are no guidelines or methods for monitoring pesticide use. Farmers overuse pesticides, hoping to increase agricultural productivity. Pesticides and insecticides are overused, diminishing the plant's natural ability to fight infections and making seeds weak, requiring pesticides and insecticides to thrive.

1. It's important to remember that plants have developed over millions of years and have developed their own defense mechanisms against pathogens, such as bitterness, anti-nutrients, poisons (some plants are poisonous to insects, animals and humans), and so on. When we eat these plants and vegetables, we gain the ability to fight pathogens. As a result, your grandmother advised you to eat seasonal vegetables and fruits.

2. Repeated use of herbicides, pesticides, and insecticides harms the normal microbial life in the soil. Farmers adopt these tactics for a variety of reasons, such as when the government significantly subsidizes fertilisers, to make them more accessible, or when the government supports and sets minimum prices for certain crops, leading farmers to use unethical practices. Another cause could be basic supply and demand, with farmers being influenced by buyer behavior, let me explain; the market is being driven by our desire to purchase the best-looking vegetables and meat. If farmers' do not fulfil aesthetic criteria, they are rejected by wholesalers or businesses. For example, vegetables and fruits are graded based on size, with high-quality goods commanding the highest price. Monoculture and contemporary farming methods such as tilling have harmed the sensitive environment. Modern crop types have resulted in

the production of grains, vegetables, and fruits abundant in calories and macronutrients, but they may also have resulted in micronutrient loss.

The current generation is gradually feeling the effects (increased fat, cancer, diabetes, and so on), and if we continue to act indiscriminately, the next generation will suffer. However, the problem is hard to solve. We are gradually approaching the point where an agricultural pandemic is imminent.

Farmers' markets, rather than supermarkets, are where I believe we should get our fruits and veggies. How can we make our food more nutritious? There is no straight forward answer.

Organic farming and food are one option that springs to mind, but further research is needed to determine whether organic agricultural methods help restore nutrients in food. Natural farming, which is slowly gaining traction in India and appears to have the potential to become a movement, could be the answer.

However, modern day food is not as healthful per gram should not deter you from consuming fruits, vegetables, and grains. As these will continue to be the best source of nutrition. We should continue to live a healthy, balanced lifestyle and be on the lookout for any indicators of malnutrition.

Another question is whether meat eaters are better off

than vegetarians and vegans. After all, livestock consumes over 60% of the area utilised for agriculture today. Keep that notion in mind. We'll go over this in further detail in the following chapter.

Chapter 5

Food–You are what you eat!

Chapter 5 – Food: You are what you eat!

The culinary culture and consumer choices have transformed at an unparalleled rate in the last few decades. The diversity of cuisine available now was unheard of a few decades ago, and it still perplexes your grandma, who cannot conceive of eating the food you do today. Your grandmothers and great grandmothers did not have access to the vast selection of food that exists now, where an Asian can eat a western diet and an American can easily access Asian cuisine. Your grandmother does not know what you eat nowadays. Even if you persuade her and force her to eat a few morsels, she will struggle to digest the meal and will moan incessantly. Her diet has always been straightforward, efficient, and nutritious. With all the confusion around food and our way of life, we are more perplexed than ever.

I believe we are victims of rapid urbanization, industrialization in which the industry has grown larger than the consumer, with a nexus to politicians in which Governments have deliberately and willingly turned a blind eye to the alarming rate of ailments driven solely by the food industry, marketing gimmickry in which gullible customers are coaxed into buying, and even so-called balanced and dubious marketing claims that deceive knowledgeable people.

Look at the labels. Each macronutrient is at odds with another; high fat vs low fat, high protein vs low carb, high fat vs low carb, low fat vs low card vs high protein, low fat and low cholesterol, and so on. There has been an intentional attempt to confuse consumers by making unsubstantiated, unconfirmed, and unfounded statements in order to fool consumers and maximize corporate profits.

The most ardent supporters of a low-fat diet have failed terribly in combating diabetes, obesity, and heart disease.

Acceptance is the first step towards transformation. We understand that the world is changing and will continue to change; customer behavior and preferences are continuously changing, as are companies' responses to it. We don't seem to have as much time as our grandparents did. With rising urbanization, modern work culture, families moving to silos from the nucleus, easy access to ready-to-eat food and foods with extended shelf lives, I would do you an injustice if I suggested you go into hibernation like a monk and eat food your grandparents had every day. Times have changed, and so have tastes. The Question is, how do you make sense of this chaos, how do you maintain mental clarity in such settings, and where do you begin?

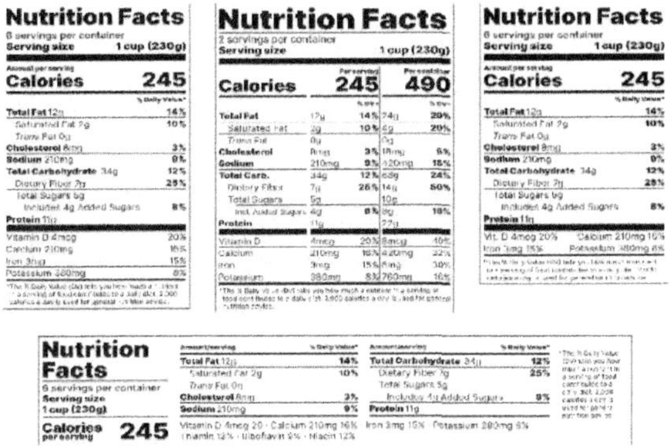

Nutrition Facts

Serving size 1 cup (230g)

Calories 245

(nutrition labels shown)

Let's begin with food labelling. I've discussed my concerns regarding food labelling in previous chapters as well. With infinite aisles of fat free, sugar free, healthy, vegan, no added sugar, low fat, natural, gut friendly bacteria, wholegrain, multigrain, and other appealing labels to fool you, discerning and making sense of labels appears herculean.

As food administrators are continuously issuing new laws and industry is continually discovering ways to work around the rules, the goal of food labels is to deceive customers and the intent of labels is to teach people to make calculated judgements.

Labels are supposed to lead the buyer, yet they invariably wind up being deceptive because labels contain carefully constructed wording designed to deceive even the most intelligent consumer. The Problem is that we are hard-wired to make split-second decisions, and businesses are well aware of this!

You're up against a multibillion-dollar industry that understands a thing or two about psychological manipulation. Firms hire and compensate food engineers handsomely to create irresistibly appealing and addicting food that encourages repeat purchases. After all, they want you to purchase more and more frequently.

The sophisticated blend of fat, sugar, salt, flavor enhancing additives, texture, and mouthfeel, where you get the same taste each bite, is exactly engineered to tap your brain's rewarding systems and entice you into making repeated purchases with the purpose of creating a conditioned behavior.

In retrospect, we become unconsciously attuned to the taste of a particular brand, for example, which ketchup brand do you frequently purchase or what is the first name that comes to mind when I say chocolate, biscuit, etc.? Brands have conditioned or trained you for loyalty where you buy their products again and again.

All said and done, you may feel obliged to buy, and if you do, here are a few tips and tricks to help you understand the labels and make the informed judgments that policymakers intended:

1. Mindful purchasing- We are hard-wired to make split-second decisions. We act differently based on our mental state. For example, if we are stressed on the day of shopping, we may choose food that provides immediate gratification. Your child throwing constant tantrums in the grocery store influences your purchasing decisions. The solution is attentive purchasing rather than mindless purchasing. Take a deep breath and a step back. Allow a few seconds (or more) before placing it in the shopping basket. Remember, *if in doubt, hold back and come back later.*

2. It is vital to note that the corporation has spent a substantial amount of money on an appealing label; therefore, when you come across an attractive label, think carefully.

3. There are always two sides to the label- The front label (less regulated) will always fool you with words like low fat, less sugar, high fiber, digestive, no sugar, free range, and so on, because here is where companies pour their marketing dollars, but what matters is the back label. Never buy a product based just on its front label. The back label always shows the policymakers' aim.

Each serving (150g) contains

Energy 1046kJ 250kcal	Fat 3.0g	Saturates 1.3g	Sugars 34g	Salt 0.9g
	LOW	LOW	HIGH	MED
13%	4%	7%	38%	15%

of an adult's reference intake
Typical values (as sold) per 100g:697kJ/167kcal

4. Serving size- The first thing you'll notice is that the listing on the back label is for the serving size rather than the entire container. For example, the serving size for corn flakes could be 100 grams, whereas the serving size for biscuits could be 28 grams, or two biscuits. If a label states 400 KJ, it may not be for the full box, and you should multiply it several times to get the actual box numbers.

5. A few techniques that companies use: Sugar is listed as the last component. Isn't this deception? It mentions vegetable oil, there is no sign of the composition of oils. Would you buy if the label said palm or soy oil? Guess what, palm oil is the world's most widely consumed vegetable oil. whether palm oil is safe is not the question. The key question is whether you will use palm oil in your regular cooking? The question, of course, answers itself.

6. Trans fat- We already know trans-fat is bad for your health. Certain policymakers permit businesses to round off trans-fat. For example, if trans-fat is 0.45 grams per serving, firms may label trans-fat as zero. You should multiply the trans-fat for the entire package. They outwit both customers and policymakers! in some countries, policymakers are now requiring corporations to provide more information, such as if hydrogenated oil is used in the ingredients section. The print is sometimes so small that it is easy to

miss.

7.   Carbohydrates, Sugars, and Fibers-Most countries now have rigorous standards in place to display carbs and fibers on packages. However, corporations have found a way around this by using maltodextrin in their products, which functions as a volume enhancer in processed foods and improves the flavor and texture of the dish. Maltodextrin is a starch, not a resistant starch; it is also not classed as sugar. It is added to total carbohydrate amounts although it behaves and processes in the body similar to sugar, with a GI higher than sugar and being worse than sugar.

8.   Companies know also that some consumers are knowledgeable, and guess what they have manufactured? Resistant maltodextrin, which allegedly behaves like resistant starch and is labelled as fiber. Resistant maltodextrin is a chemically manufactured fiber; but, because it is a recent introduction, there has been little research on it, and until policymakers wake up, firms will ride the wave and take you for a ride as well!

9.   The unholy whole grain - The simplest approach to deceive people is to put whole grain on the front label. Remember when I mentioned pulverised food? The Problem is that the whole grain does not exclude ultra-processed grain. Then they released 100% whole grain food. While the whole grain included is 100% whole grain, it also contains ultra-processed grain. The issue with

whole grains is that if the bread is 100% whole grain, it does not swell and does not have the same texture or taste. Companies add chemicals, flavor and texture enhancers, and other ingredients to make it look and taste the same. Always inspect the rear label as an extra precaution.

10. Shelf life- We all know that natural food has a shorter shelf life than packaged food. Natural foods deteriorate because of oxidative damage (damage caused by oxygen exposure) and spoiling caused by microbial development. The flavor, texture, and odor of natural food vary over time can spoil in a matter of days two weeks.

Oxidation is a biological chain reaction that occurs in the presence of oxygen and leads to food degradation, flavor changes, texture changes, and so on, eventually diminishing the shelf life (apple slices turning brown are because of oxidative stress).

Your grandparents were well aware of this, and historically, humans have utilised a variety of natural techniques of preserving food, such as salt in pickles, sugar in marmalade, vinegar, fermentation in yoghurt, and so on. Unfortunately, these strategies are difficult to apply to a pack of biscuits or a loaf of bread.

Food scientists have developed a variety of preservatives (chemical compositions) that are added to food to increase shelf life, keep flavor, texture, and so on. There are two ways to increase shelf life: one by adding acids to prevent microbial growth, where acids make the food inhospitable to the microbes, and the other by adding anti-oxidant chemicals to prevent oxidative damage.

Policymakers think that preservatives in modest concentrations do not harm humans and have restricted their use. Although human study is in its early stages, few studies have found that this causes harm to humans. Consumption of sodium benzoate (anti-microbial) typically found in ketchup, for example, causes hyperactivity in people.

While our forefathers' preservation techniques have been around for generations, the use of preservatives in packaged food is recent (30-40 years); it will take time to determine the true impact of preservatives on humans. Until then, I would advise "tread carefully." I recognize that eliminating the consumption of preserved foods is impossible. However, we may always try to limit our usage and use our judgement wisely.

Now that we've learned a few things about foods to avoid, let's look at foods to include in our diets and why they're important.

We may have gotten far from our roots because of

ready-to-eat food and the ease with which food is available in restaurants around us. The next paragraphs are an attempt to return you to your roots and potentially improve your behavior!

Germination and fermentation:

As a prelude to this topic, let's talk about seeds and anti-nutrients. Seeds are a natural wonder that has existed from the beginning of time. A seed is a living embryo (similar to an egg) and a reservoir of macro and micronutrients. It delicately stores micro and macro nutrients to help the seed sprout and spread life. The genesis of seeds is not to provide us with nourishment, but to provide all the life-giving elements for the next generation of plant, where given the correct environment (water, temperature, etc.), the seed will spring to life and give rise to a new plant. A seed can stay dormant for hundreds or even thousands of years under certain conditions before sprouting if given the correct habitat.

As an example, we know seeds contain carbohydrate, protein, fat, and micronutrients. Seeds also contain anti-nutrients, such as phytate, polyphenols, Oxalate, Enzyme inhibitors, Lectins, and so on.

Let's inspect anti-nutrients before we go into fermentation and germination. Listed below are a few notable anti-nutrients.

Phytic acid or phytate-

We can find Phytic acid in a variety of foods, including seeds and pulses. Phytates are formed when Phytic acid binds to minerals in the seed. Because we lack enzymes to dissolve phytates, the activity of binding hinders the human digestive system from readily absorbing nourishment, and hence, phytic acid is labelled as an antinutrient. Phytic acid, in a limited quantity, has cancer-fighting capabilities. We can find Phytic acid in beans, seeds, and nuts (Almonds have the highest amount of phytic acid).

Our forefathers discovered many ways to reduce the impact of phytic acid, including cooking, soaking in water, using it with garlic and onion, removing the outer skin, germination, and fermentation, all of which have been found to reduce the phytate content in the food, particularly germination and fermentation. This also increases the bioavailability of micronutrients.

Tannins: [53]These are found in many plant foods, such as tea and pulses. Tannins are both a blessing and a curse because they hinder protein precipitation and can interfere with vitamin/mineral absorption. Tannins are also recognized for their anti-cancer and anti-microbial properties. According to research, excessive tannin consumption may be harmful to our health; however, moderate tannin consumption may be healthy.

Oxalates: We typically find oxalates in leafy greens

(such as Spinach), nuts, and seeds. Oxalates bound to calcium, limiting calcium and nutrient absorption.[54]

Lectins[55]: These are possibly insecticidal and part of plants' natural defense against insects and pests. We can discover lectins in pulses, which are commonly available. Lectins can obstruct iron, phosphorus, and zinc absorption.

Saponins: we find Saponins in pulses. They give bitter taste. plants developed this adaption to protect their seeds from insects and herbivores. They may impair protein absorption, as well as vitamin and mineral absorption.

Plants and seeds that contain anti-nutrients should not be avoided. Although there are some limiting considerations, naturally occurring poisons have never been a hazard to people. Our bodies effectively eliminate toxins. In fact, the bitterness in bitter guard, fenugreek and other dietary items, caffeine in coffee, oxalates in Spinach, and phylates on almond skins are harmful to us in high doses, moderate and balanced nutrition do not appear to be harmful. Through evolution, humans have developed to effectively isolate and eliminate certain toxins. However, the reality remains that they hinder and limit nutrient absorption.

Our forefathers devised brilliant techniques to mitigate the effects of these anti-nutrients, and they have gone a long way toward increasing the nutritional density of foods.

For example, we know that oxalates (found in Spinach) hinder calcium absorption, while calcium absorbability improves dramatically when ingested with dairy. We always serve spinach with cottage cheese in some parts of India. This cannot be a coincidence. Our forefathers intuitively understood the benefits of dairy and Spinach. There are several methods for increasing absorbability, such as soaking, wherein they soak and rinse pulses before to cooking, effectively cleaning out water soluble anti-nutrients from the skin's surface. Another method is to cook the pulses. However, soaking and boiling can only diminish anti-nutrients to a certain level and never significantly. Cooking may destroy certain vitamins and hence does not deliver entire nutritional benefits.

Fermentation and germination are excellent methods for preserving imbedded nutrients, breaking down anti-nutrients, unlocking, unmasking, and boosting nutrient bioavailability, and improving nutrition. Fermented foods have been consumed throughout human history. Fermentation has been practised in various forms by many cultures all over the world.

Fermentation is the oldest known technique of food processing in which food is broken down and processed into a more appetizing form. The earliest reported fermentation dates back to 10,000 BCE.

Fermentation is a process in which microbes break food down such as bacteria, yeast, and others. These microorganisms are naturally present and require the correct environment to reproduce and thrive.

Throughout history, people have fermented and consumed a wide variety of foods, including vegetables, cereals, legumes, meat, drinks, dairy, and even bones.

I could claim with considerable certainty that your ancestors ate fermented food, regardless of where you live, what culture you belong to, or whether you are a vegetarian or a non-vegetarian.

A few notable fermentation processes used around the world include:

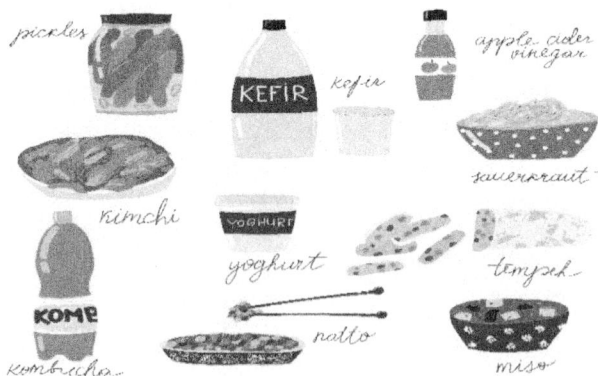

1. Yeast used in the bread-making process, your ancestors had found a way to ferment food they eat and raise the dough;

2. People throughout the world consume yoghurt or curd, cheese, and kefir.
3. Beverages such as beer and wine, for example.
4. Kimchi, Doenjang, and other Korean fermented dishes, Natto/ Miso in Japan, Tempeh in Indonesia, Nem Chua in Vietnam, Douchi/ Doubanjiang/Mianchi in China, Bagoong in the Philippines, and Idli/ Dosa/ Dhokla/ Jalebi/ Kadi in India.
5. Injera, Togwa/Mahewu/Mabundu, Furundu/Ogiri, Garri, Kenkey, and Dawadawa, to mention a few African foods.
6. In the American continent, there is Sourdough Bread, Poi, Atole agrio, and curtido.
7. Kefir, Sauerkraut, Smetana, Kiviak, Hakarl, and Kvass throughout Europe.
8. Apple cider vinegar

What is fermentation?

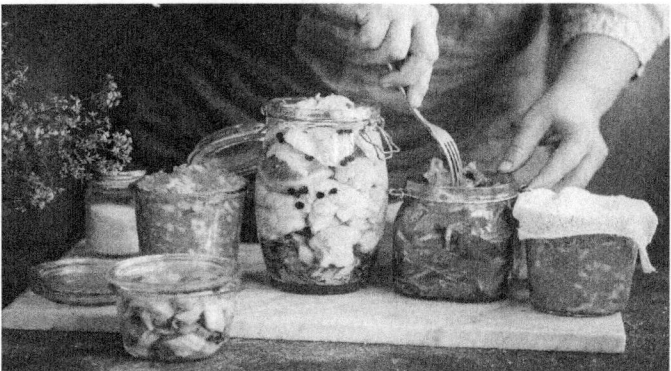

Fermentation is a process in which we either add

microbe (for example, yeast to bread or Kefir culture to milk to make Kefir) or use a mother culture from previous fermentation (for example, yoghurt) or let nature take its course, in which microbes present in the food, container, or hand of the person fermenting act as a culture.

Microbes break down food by consuming sections of it and releasing byproducts (such as carbon dioxide, which makes the bread bulge).

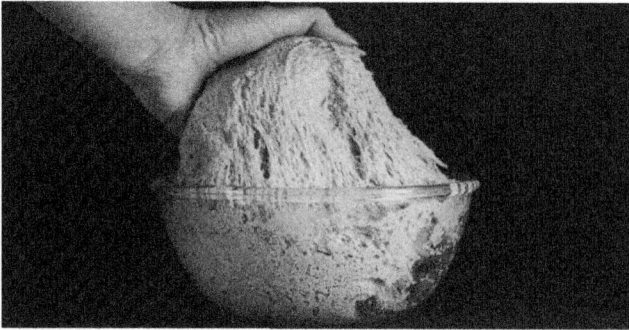

Fermentation was used as a food preservation technique around the world, making it more delicious, palatable, and so on, this is not the only reason our forefathers took the time and effort to prepare it; our forefathers secretly knew of the immense benefits we could derive from fermented foods.

For millennia, humans and bacteria have had a symbiotic connection in which both have helped one other, and this has formed human civilization.

Passion and affection for the fermentation process, where the mother culture is lovingly conserved and repeated for generations, is the tether for all fermenting cultures.

Fermentation, for example, is so deeply ingrained in Japanese culture it has become more of an art and way of life, and fermented foods such as miso, soy sauce, mirin, and sake are utilised in everyday cooking. There is a mountain of evidence showing fermentation is extremely helpful to humans, here are a few of the advantages:[56]

1. Alteration in carbohydrate content. Microbes require energy to grow and multiply. Glucose is one of their energy sources. Fermentation causes chemical reactions that break down carbs into their constituents. As a result, the concentration of glucose decreases as microorganisms use it for energy. The starch composition has also changed. Have you ever noticed curd/yogurt being sweet for the first 24-48 hours and then turning sour after a few days, or wines having distinct sweet or tartness, or why sour bread is called that? And as a result of microbial waste, carbon dioxide is released (bubbles in bread, carbonation in beer) or acids are created (natural ethanol in beer). Nature is performing reverse engineering and working its magic. These mechanisms result in a relative decrease in carbohydrate. Consumption of fermented food

shall surely aid in weight management.

2. Protein availability- Protein bioavailability and digestibility may be enhanced, resulting in easier absorption by the intestines. Plant protein, for example, is less digestible than animal protein. Protein bioavailability is increased by fermentation.

3. Minerals-Fermentation boosts the bioavailability of many minerals, including potassium, magnesium, iron, calcium, zinc, and phosphorus. This is likely because of the breaking or loosening of carbohydrate and protein chains where the seed encases or holds certain minerals together making them unavailable for absorption and fermentation breaks or unlocks certain anti-nutrients such as oxalates and phytates resulting in an increase in mineral bioavailability.

4. Anti-nutrients[57]: Fermentation can break down phylates and lectins through microbial activity. Fermentation, for example, has been proven to remove nearly all lectins in lentils. Natural bread fermentation has been showed to drastically reduce phylates (although not eliminate phylates; remember, phylates in moderate quantities are beneficial to humans).

5. It is only recently that research has discovered that having a wide variety of live cultured fermented foods in our diet can have a tremendous impact on the gut microbiota, increasing gut micro diversity and improving general health and wellbeing.

6. Fermented foods can stimulate the gut microbiota,

resulting in a healthier mix of microorganisms and stronger intestine walls, ultimately reducing leaky gut.

7. Fermentation causes the release of some phytochemical (byproducts of fermentation) that have antioxidant and anti-inflammatory properties, according to the study.

8. Consuming fermented foods increases the number of friendly bacteria while decreasing the number of unfavorable bacteria.

9. The bacteria in fermented foods speed up your metabolism and help you lose weight. As discussed in the previous chapter, fermented foods will evoke a pleasant mood, lower anxiety, and make you feel good in terms of gut brain cross talk.

Louis Pasteur invented Pasteurization in 1860, a method that involves heating food (fermented or otherwise) to a specific temperature in order to kill microorganisms. All canned food in supermarkets is pasteurized, and even so-called fermented food is pasteurized, killing all bacteria, including healthy ones. Although pasteurization has saved many lives, it also nearly destroyed the microbial variety.

With the industrialization of food, it has become nearly impossible to discriminate between the good and the bad; for example, bread from your local bakery or grocery store practically never employs live yeast. They only use baking powder and baking soda, the flour they use is ultra-processed, so even the purported benefits are negated. Due to mass manufacturing, natural fermentation, in which mother culture was kept and reused, is a lost art; nowadays, firms employ synthetic yeast, baking powder, and baking soda for dough levelling and bread making.

It is time to abandon processed and canned foods in favour of fermented foods with live cultures or even cooked fermented foods, which will cause a significant increase in mineral and vitamin bioavailability. It is difficult to prescribe a specific fermentation procedure because it depends on geographical region and cultural preferences.

You may need to think back on the fermented foods your grandparents used to eat and instill them in your daily diet.

However, yoghurt or curd is the simplest way to get probiotics into your diet, and studies have shown that eating yogurt/curd may help you lose weight.

It is important to remember that you should consume food that has not been pasteurized, contains living cultures, and contains no added sugar. Lactic Acid Bacillus (LCA), the bacteria that causes curdling, can only grow at a specific temperature. if you live in a tropical area, curd/yogurt is easily accessible/available, and you can curdle it at home with ease. It may be tough to inoculate and ferment if you live in chilly weather. Here, you could look into portable yoghurt producing devices, which are now reasonably priced.

Let's look at some other foods that can help or supplement your efforts to maintain a healthy weight. The aim is to reduce your intake of processed foods and shift to healthier options while maintaining the diet you've been following for years. The ideas in the following paragraphs are practical, simple to practice, and easy to absorb. You can experiment with these ideas or ingredients, continue or cease at your leisure, and these have no negative side effects.

Germination (Sprouting):

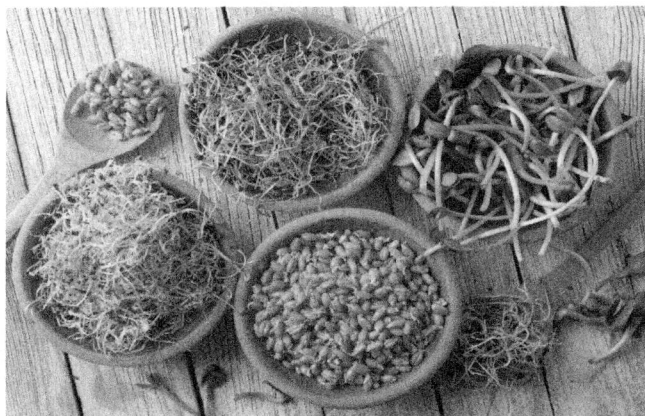

My younger brother was born when I was about eight years old. We weaned him between the ages of 6 and 12 months, and my mother introduced him to malts (not the malt used in alcoholic beverages!).

I didn't understand malting until I went to my grandparents' house and saw my grandmother going through an elaborate malting procedure in which[58] she chose a few grains, washed them, submerged them in water overnight, and let them sprout.

I marveled as I watched the seeds transform right in front of my eyes. She would then stop the germination process by drying the sprouting seeds in a hot, dry environment. She would next lightly roast and grind the seeds into a course powder. My brother took a few days to adjust because he had bloating issues at first, but he eventually came to enjoy the malt.

When I questioned my grandma why she was going through such trouble, she explained it was nutritious for my brother and simple to digest. In fact, we drank malts made by our grandmother until we were in our twenties. Malt was our go-to morning beverage.

With ready-to-eat infant formulae on supermarket shelves, the technique of malting for children has slowly vanished. Our grandmother insisted we continue to eat it even during adolescence and maturity, when the components changed based on age group; we did not listen to our grandmother.

Sprouting and malting have been around for a long time; sprouts were part of the eastern cuisine, where they were eaten alone or as part of a salad, and malts were part of our normal food.

It has gained popularity in western countries over the last two to three decades. Our grandmothers were wiser than us. They knew what was best for us and went to tremendous lengths to keep the art alive.

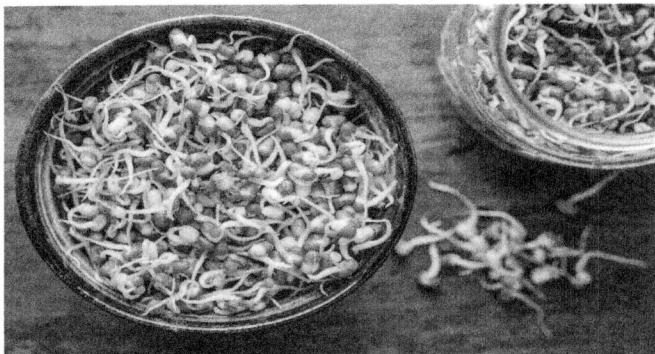

We frequently ignore nature's wonders, and it is not part of our school curriculum. Because Grains and seeds are so common, we often ignore their formation. Seeds are an evolutionary marvel that we are unaware of since we take them for granted. Let us digress for a moment and use the egg as an example. We all know that a chicken egg is high in nourishment and, with the proper temperature and care, can hatch into a chick. As a result, an egg (yolk and albumin to the naked eye) has all the ingredients for life. The yolk and albumin, for example, are enclosed in a hard shell with pores for air permeability; the yolk is rich in vitamins, minerals, glucose, protein, calcium, and cholesterol; all the vital materials required for life are delicately balanced and wrapped in an egg.

To use a comparable analogy, a seed is not different from an egg. A seed is an embryonic plant that forms after fertilization (akin to animal reproduction), and it comprises three key parts: the seed coat (the outer skin), the embryo, and the endosperm. The earliest forms of plants, roots, stems, and leaves are found in embryos. The embryo is nutritionally packed, containing protein and other vitamins, as well as a small quantity of carbs.

Endosperm contains carbohydrates, protein, fat, and a few micronutrients. The seed coat is mostly fiber with a little protein and lipids. When the seed germinates, the endosperm kick-starts the embryo by causing changes in starch production, fat formation, and transferring certain important nutrients to the embryo. the embryo is where the plant develops. The plant grows from the embryo because of genetic and epigenetic alterations. During this time, the seed undergoes metamorphosis, which causes substantial changes in both macro and micronutrients.

Certain micronutrients that were previously bio unavailable (because of anti-nutrients) undergo modifications and become bio available.

Carbohydrates and fats undergo modifications, with carbohydrates providing energy to the developing embryo and fats providing enzymes for embryo development. Protein undergoes structural changes to assist plants in sprouting and growing.

Seeds contain enzyme inhibitors, which prevent the formation of important enzymes in the stomach. Germination has the potential to neutralise [59]these inhibitors and ensure enzyme release.

The question that requires an answer is, how does sprouting assist us get the most benefit, and why am I emphasizing the relevance of sprouted seeds in our diet?

Here are a few examples:

1. Carbohydrate - Carbohydrate is found[60] in legumes and grains and is used to provide energy to the growing embryo, carbohydrates are broken down and transformed into simple sugars during the early phase to supply energy to the seeds. During this process, enzymatic modifications take place. This improves digestibility, since simple sugars are easier to digest. It's no surprise that sprouted seeds are included in newborn formulae. What stands out is the sprouting period; as the sprout erupts and expands, there is a rise in fiber content that ranges from 100% to 500%. This is possibly one reason your gut microbiome enjoys sprouts. This will also result in satiety and a full feeling, and as a result, we will be less hungry for a longer period.

2. Proteins - Proteins are required for plant growth. A seed requires protein as an impulse for stem and root growth from the standpoint of the plant. This is critical during the early stages, since the immature

embryo may not produce protein on its own. During germination, the protein composition changes to provide protein for the developing embryo. The modifications in protein composition make it easier for humans to digest. Protein content increases significantly with extended sprouting time.

Protein quality and quantity rise dramatically, according to research. So much so that the protein content of pulses exceeds that of meat in terms of quality. Certain anti-nutrients impair our ability to absorb protein. Sprouting lowers the impact of these anti-nutrients.

3. Minerals-Germination starts enzymatic activities that effectively suppress the influence of anti-nutrients (such as Phytate) that bind to minerals and impede nutrient absorption. Mineral content increases dramatically during germination, according to research. Seeds can also absorb minerals from water, which has been proven in a few experiments to boost iron and calcium levels.

4. Vitamins - The sprouts have a considerable[61] increase in Vitamin B and Vitamin C content.

5. Fats-At the start of germination, the seed's fat content increases. this makes sense because the seed is preparing for a growth spurt and the chemical composition is changing, resulting in a minor increase in fat. However, as time passes, the seedling utilizes fat and transforms it into energy, resulting

in fat loss.

6. No chemicals- The sprouts develop directly in front of your eyes and require no soil. They don't require any particular containers or medium to grow; you can use any utensil to produce sprouts, and they don't take up much space. As part of the sprouting process, you rinse and wash the seeds repeatedly, cleaning away any pesticides or toxins.

7. Rinsing and washing also removes any anti-nutrients on the seed's surface, providing you with the cleanest and most efficient source of energy. It takes a few days for a fruit or vegetable to reach the grocery store shelf, and another few days to a week for it to reach your plate. Sprouts are ready in seconds. On your kitchen counter, you have access to fresh food.

8. Anti-cancer properties-Sulforaphane (SFN), a phytonutrient present in sprouts of cruciferous plants such as broccoli and cauliflower, offers incredible health advantages. Professor Talalay [62]and his colleagues discovered that broccoli sprouts provide excellent cancer prevention.

Carcinogens in food are compounds that quietly infiltrated our systems because of the industrial revolution. It was discovered that these sprouts stimulate carcinogen detoxification enzymes. SFN is unique in that it only targets cancer cells and not healthy cells (also called apoptosis). Because the SFN present in these sprouts is so concentrated, all you need is a small bit to reap the advantages.

It may be questioned why we should ingest cruciferous plant sprouts rather than the cruciferous vegetable itself. Scientists discovered SFN in cruciferous vegetables; however, the concentration is reduced when compared to cruciferous seed sprouts, which are 20 to 50 times more effective than their vegetable equivalent.

In order to reap the benefits of cruciferous vegetables, they should be ingested as soon as possible because the concentration of SFN gradually decreases with time, with up to 80% loss in the first 10 days. Sprouts have a short shelf life and must be consumed as soon as possible. We all know that the cruciferous vegetables accessible these days are riddled with chemicals, and we have little choice but to wash and boil them before eating, resulting in cancer fighting chemicals to leak out into the water as many of the cancer fighting chemicals are water soluble.

As a result, cruciferous sprouts can prevent and control cancer. Still not convinced? SFN has been discovered to have neuroprotective characteristics, which are employed in the treatment of traumatic brain damage, Parkinson's disease, Alzheimer's disease, and certain Autism spectrum disorders. Certain molecules in SFN are beneficial against a variety of allergies.

SFN has anti-inflammatory characteristics and is useful in the prevention of asthma, colitis, arthritis, and other diseases. SFN is also reported to lower cholesterol and prevent non-alcoholic fatty liver disease (one of the obesity conditions). Broccoli sprouts are high in soluble fiber and Chromium, both of which are good for diabetics.

9. Finally, SFN and cruciferous sprouts may have anti-aging benefits when combined.

10. Sprouting is a low-cost, less labor-intensive method, all you need is a container and a few edible seeds to get started. Once you've mastered the technique, you can rinse and repeat. When a seed sprouts, its weight increases substantially, this is attributed to increased fiber content because of photosynthesis and water absorption; the increase in volume helps with satiety. Sprouts do not need to be cooked (but larger seeds may require cooking). However, each person is unique. Start little and build up slowly. Sprouts are more filling and provide more energy/nutrients per cup. As sprouts increase in volume, it is more filling and bingeing sprouts is never a possibility.

11. They're high in fiber and protein; the nutrients are accessible and easily absorbed by the colon; the gut bacteria loves them; and they'll eventually help you lose weight. You may easily incorporate sprouts into any of your daily diet, whether it's salads, curry, or snacks; the choices are limitless.

12. Sprouts are a nutritional powerhouse that even omnivores should include in their diet instead of ultra-processed carbohydrates. It is never too late to eat fiber and sprouts if you are a carnivore.

13. Unlike cooked food, sprouts must be chewed and churned many times in the mouth before consumption. the act of masticating not only ensures that the food is properly mixed with oral enzymes, but it also naturally prevents us from bingeing by making us feel satiated with smaller portion sizes and staying satiated for longer because sprouts are high in complex carbohydrates.

    The result is weight loss!

14. Sprouts improve and supply key vitamins and minerals such as magnesium, potassium, calcium, protein, Vitamin B and Vitamin C, which improves bone health, delays ageing, enhances immunity, and promotes hair development. You could grow your own multivitamin on your kitchen counter with sprouts

    It also aids in the prevention of artery thickening, lowering the risk of heart disease. Sprouts have a low glycemic index. Sprouting is a lifestyle change, the more you sprout, the more you like it and will finally fall in love with it.

15. With sprouts, you are the creator because you see life emerge right before your eyes from a dormant,

unassuming seed. You nurture the seeds for a few days to search and wonder at how they mature.

Sometimes I peak in the jar curiously (and sometimes often) to see how much they've grown and to remove any unsprouted ones. You will never have a more fulfilling experience than sprouting. The seed has come to life right in front of your eyes; you have nursed it the entire time and are confident that it is in its purest form, free of any contaminants.

16. The pleasure you gain from sprouting is enormous, and it pushes you to do more. you will appreciate the beauty of nature as you study and grow in sprouting! Why not give it a shot? I guarantee you will not be sorry.

17. In terms of which sprouts to consume and how much to consume, it is always best to consume sprouts in moderation as part of a balanced diet and not to overdo it. It's also a good idea to start small and gradually expand, and to have a variety of seeds in sprouts.

For example, pulse sprouts are high in protein, cruciferous sprouts have a plethora of health benefits, flax seed sprouts are high in omega-3 and excellent source of healthy fat, and so on.

Millets:

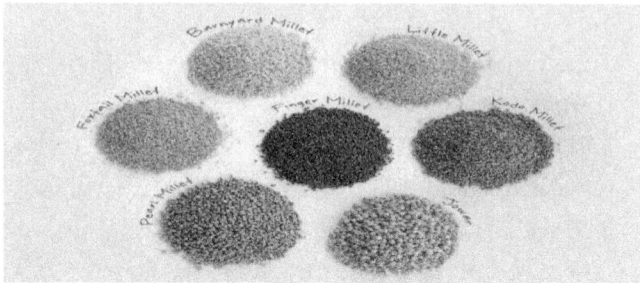

The world is currently divided into wheat, maize or corn, and rice, with these grain kinds being a staple all throughout the world. This was not the case half a century ago, when millets played an important part in human and agricultural evolution. Millets are a tiny group of grasses that formed part of the regular human diet. Now, millet is consumed rarely in India and many other regions of the world because of the dominance of other grass species.

Millets were previously commonly consumed, according to researchers who unearthed them in archaeological sites in China, India, and Europe. Porso millet, barnyard millet, foxtail millet, and other millets are examples. Ironically, millets are used as bird feed in the United States and a few European countries (have you ever seen a fat bird?). However, it was and still is consumed daily in areas of India, China, South America, Russia, and parts of Europe.

Millet is consumed as a whole grain, so, unlike wheat

varieties, the fiber, bran, and endosperm are not separated. Millet, like any other grain, contains carbohydrates. It is notable for being an excellent source of protein, complex carbohydrates, and micronutrients. Unlike wheat, corn, and rice, this is one of the few grains that is not mass produced, it is a resilient grass that can withstand extreme conditions and is resistant to insect and disease infestations. As a result, when compared to rice and wheat, the need for insecticides and pesticides is comparatively low. Millets are also gluten-free, giving them an advantage over wheat. Millets have gained popularity and are now appearing on shop shelves.

Although more expensive than wheat and rice, they are worth the extra money given the benefits. Here are some advantages of millets and why you should incorporate them in your daily diet:

1. Fiber-Millets are high in soluble and insoluble fiber. Fiber can account for up to 10% of millet. Fiber has already proven to be beneficial.
2. Resistant starch - Millets are high in Resistant starch[63]. Millets have 20-30% slowly digested starch and 25-30% resistant starch. Millets have the most resistant starch for any cereal. According to research, finger millet starches are resistant to digestive enzymes due to their stiff starch granule structure when compared to rice. When compared to commonly used rice and wheat starches, Kodo

millet starch has a high RS.

3. Micronutrients-As previously said, millets are drought tolerant and may flourish in arid weather. Millets are less sensitive to common pest infestations and do not require extensive farming techniques to produce and harvest. Grown on potentially healthy soils, they are a rich source of micronutrients.

4. Low GI- Millets have a GI of between 50 and 65. This amounts to around 40% less than white rice and ultra-processed wheat.

5. Niacin, Vitamin B6, folic acid, calcium, iron, potassium, and other micronutrients are abundant in millet.

6. Preliminary research shows that millet eating lowers blood glucose, cholesterol, and triglyceride levels, as well as inflammation.

7. A recently completed study found64 that diabetics who eat millet had a 10%-15% decrease in blood glucose levels. Millet has showed promise in lowering blood glucose levels. However, incorporating millet into your daily diet may be difficult.

Here are a few ideas for incorporating this into your daily diet:

1. Supplement with rice-depending on how you use rice, you can use millet whole or ground. With steamed rice, all you need to do is soak millet in

warm water for a few hours before steaming and cook it alongside rice in any proportion (50:50, 75:25 etc.).

2. Use in place of cooked white rice - This is an acquired taste that you can develop. All that is required is to soak millet in warm water before cooking. If substituting millet for rice is difficult, alternate rice and millet.

3. Add to wheat- Try adding ground millet in the desired proportion to wheat-based breads. However, the wheat bread may change from its original taste, flavor, and texture. It could be a learned taste that takes a few days or meals. However, this is a step in the right direction, and your taste buds/mind will adjust without you even recognizing it.

ACV (Apple Cider Vinegar) -

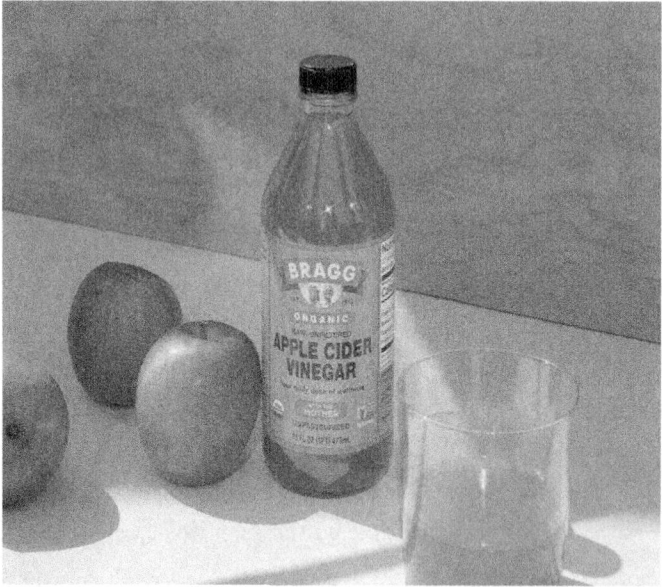

The bad news is that when you search ACV on the internet, it is marketed as a miracle cure for instant weight loss and other amazing health advantages. Quick weight loss is a myth, weight loss and maintenance are a long and laborious process that requires you to believe in and instill the right methods rather than looking for short remedies. Another concern among dietitians is the apparent lack of scientific study on ACV. As you will see in the following paragraphs, there is enough information to persuade and encourage you to incorporate ACV into your diet.

ACV has been a popular family staple for many

millennia and is mentioned in many ancient literatures around the world. ACV has historically been used to treat arthritis, diabetes, acne, hair loss, weight loss, bowel movement disorders, killing bacteria in the colon, and, believe it or not, as a deodorant!

While people utilised it as a common home item and as a medication, it wasn't until 1822 that Christian Persoon discovered bacteria are responsible for Vinegar creation. He determined that Acetobacter aceti, a bacterium, was in charge of vinegar creation. ACV is fermented apple juice that is first fermented to alcohol using yeast.

Acetobacter aceti, a naturally occurring bacteria, then neutralizes the alcohol to produce acetic acid. ACV contains about 5-6% acetic acid, which gives it its strong pungent odor. There are other acids and bacteria, but acetic acid stands out. ACV is said to offer many advantages; a few notable weight control advantages are listed below:

Insulin Inhibition-We know from the insulin chapter that insulin may mess with our weight, especially in persons who have insulin resistance.

To recap, the more insulin we have in our blood, the less likely we are to lose weight, because insulin promotes fat production and inhibits fat burning.

Acetic acid has been found in studies[65]to suppress

insulin production, where particular receptors triggered by acetic acid instruct or prevent the pancreas from making too much insulin. Scientists [66]have also discovered a considerable decrease in the GI of foods ingested with Vinegar.

No surprise that we use ACV as a salad dressing in western culture; vinegar and pickled foods are common in Japanese daily staple diets.

According to one study, individuals consumed fewer calories on days when they consumed vinegar. A Japanese study found that vinegar consumption lowers body fat ([67],[68]) body weight, and serum triglyceride levels in Japanese individuals. Over the course of three months, the patients in the research dropped approximately 1-2 kilograms.

Remember that while this may not appear to be much at first glance, but we can derive considerable benefit when combined with a well-balanced diet. I am confident that with a well-balanced diet, we will see tangible results.

Personally, I've been drinking ACV for over 5 years and believe it's one reason I'm able to sustain my weight.

Digestion-ACV aids digestion by acting as an Enzyme activator and starter. In the intestines, several enzymes are dormant. Unfiltered, raw, and organic ACV includes protein strands, enzymes, and microorganisms, acting as a probiotic and instilling good intestinal microbiota. We already know that having a healthy microbiome is beneficial.

Other advantages-ACV has antipathogenic characteristics where it helps in controlling pathogens because it acts as a PH balancer in the stomach and intestines.

ACV has been found in animal research to promote heart health by lowering cholesterol and triglycerides ([69], [70] and [71]) ACV has also been shown to promote skin health and ease certain skin disorders, such as eczema, when[72] applied topically. It also helps with conditions like acid reflux.

As you can see, there are many advantages to using ACV. You can take one or two tablespoons with sufficient water before, after, or during a meal. You can also take it before bedtime, as ACV is effective at lowering fasting blood sugar levels (more on this in the fasting chapter). Please don't overdo it, and take in moderation. You can also use a straw because the acidity of ACV might damage tooth enamel.

You can mix ACV with salt, lemon juice, ginger, and other ingredients to make a salad dressing.

What to eat and what not to eat:

For the past few decades, there has been a lot of

confusion about whether humans are herbivores, carnivores, or omnivores, and what the benefits and drawbacks of these dietary patterns. Whether meat is healthy, whether a plant-based diet provides adequate nourishment, and so on?

Famously, Michael Pollan recommended his readers to "Consume food. Not excessively. Mostly plants". The Beatles' Sir James Paul McCartney famously stated, "If slaughterhouses had glass walls, we'd all be vegetarians." Humans are an odd species; we adore lambs but still eat sheep, traffic comes to a standstill when a flock of ducks cross the road but we eat ducks and its close relative chicken end up on our plates, we adore piglets but cherish pork, we love meat but don't want to see the animals suffer; would you ever confine a hen in a shoe box for its entire life and then slaughter it?

Hunger and our taste buds make us readily cross so-called ethical thresholds, and with increasing urbanization, the meat on our plate resembles a vegetable.

For thousands of years, meat has been a significant part of the human diet, providing protein, fat, micronutrients, and even energy during times of carbohydrate scarcity (such as for people in the arctic). There are arguments and research both in favour and against a meat diet.

Several studies ([73], [74], [75], [76],) have connected processed meat and red meat intake to an increased risk of heart disease. A number of research ([77], [78], [79], [80], [81], [82], [83], [84], [85]) have found conclusive evidence and a correlation between processed/red meat consumption and type 2 diabetes. It is crucial to highlight, however, that few of these studies were observational, so we should take them with a grain of salt. Given the following factors, I would be skeptical about these studies as:

1. Other contributing and underlying risk factors may exist.
2. These studies are observational; they required the participants under observation to complete questionnaires, etc.; the study is not comprehensive.
3. It is also difficult to determine if the study participants ate grass-fed (free-range) beef or processed meat.

   The reason for asking this question is that humans have been eating meat for thousands of years, and the meat they have eaten has always come from free-range animals rather than the rapidly expanding, chemically laden farm animals of recent decades.
4. The sort of meat we eat affects our risk of cancer and other diseases. There is conclusive[86] evidence that consuming processed meat causes cancer, particularly colon cancer. Hot dogs, ham, sausages, corned beef, biltong or beef jerky, canned meat, and

meat-based dishes and sauces are examples of processed meat.

5. Another reason for contemplation is to consider whether our forefathers ate meat every day and three times a day. Perhaps the answer is a resounding no. Even the most carnivorous tribes on the planet included plant-based foods into their daily diets. Every culture has a salad or a plant-based meal. Certain civilizations eat meat on some days and plant-based foods on others. During the 1900s, they reserved daily omnivore meal for the elite and affluent and were not readily available to the general population.

Even today, the world's middle and lower middle-class omnivore population has embraced plant-based cuisine. Maybe we were asking the incorrect question. The question isn't whether meat is healthy; it's whether consuming only meat and excluding plant-based foods is healthy.

Be aware that if you eat only meat or carnivorous foods, you may be deficient in certain essential nutrients, such as carbohydrates, potassium, certain vitamins, and so on.

6. Organ meats, for example, are nutrient dense and contain far more nutrients than veggies. Organ meats are often the liver, kidney, brain, and heart of an organism that was preferably grass-fed and possibly organically raised without the use of hazardous chemicals. Unfortunately, most meat consumed by the general people is muscle meat

rather than organ meat.

7. Another likely reason for a rise in cancer risk among meat users is how meat is prepared, as meat cooked at high temperatures may raise cancer risk. There is evidence that certain toxic compounds are released when meat is cooked regularly at high temperatures (such as in an oil or pan), where certain harmful chemicals may concentrate and build up on the cooking surface. High-temperature cooking, causes the creation of a chemical known as polycyclic aromatic hydrocarbons (PAHs), which has been linked to cancer (**87, 88**). It is crucial to highlight that the study on white meat (i.e., chicken) is still ambiguous, and only time will tell whether this meat is toxic and whether cooking white meat at high temperatures may have similar detrimental effects.

8. There has been a seismic shift in the meat we consume over the last many decades. Today's meat is mass produced on farms and in cages where hundreds or thousands of animals are grown in tight confines. It is estimated that over 60-70% of the 70 billion terrestrial animals produced each year in the world are reared in closed cages under intensive farming.

9. In recent years, scientists have complained about modern-day animal husbandry. Farmers and the poultry industry, for example, feed antibiotics to chickens to protect (or so they claim) them against disease. Because hens are maintained in unsanitary conditions, allowing diseases to spread quickly and

farmers are forced to feed chickens with antibiotics and reportedly lengthen the chickens' longevity. Another key reason why farmer's feed antibiotics to chicken is that it promotes growth and boosts muscle mass. In terms of weight, farm chickens are twice as large and require nearly half the time to grow as free-range hens, and antibiotics are the secret potion! Antibiotics invariably infiltrate the food chain when humans ingest them, leading to antibiotic resistance. It is estimated that over 70% of all antibiotics manufactured around the globe is given to farm animals. In the United States alone, 80% of all antibiotics manufactured are used in the livestock business. Unless the chicken is free range, all modern chicken is a hazardous cocktail of chemicals.

In terms of production and consumption, chicken is rapidly overtaking (or has already surpassed in a few nations) all other meats, including red meats.

Chicken has developed from an animal raised in small flocks for eggs and only consumed on special occasions to one that is mass-produced for its flesh, where it has become an industrialised commodity. With humble origins, the south Asian Jungle Foul (i.e., Indian native Chicken variant) has been the world ruler of human food, spanning civilizations and populations. Although humans tamed hens 7000 to 10,000 years ago, they rarely produced chickens for meat and never on the massive scale that we see today. Hens were formerly free-range backyard scavengers bred only for their eggs. One of the primary reasons for rearing chicken was for sport's i.e., cockfighting. Unlike today, chicken was not commercially available during the nineteenth century; humans did not intend to raise chickens for meat; farmers originally raised chicken in their backyard for eggs, the hen would be culled when it lost fertility, and the cocks would be consumed/sold when the herd had many harems.

Yes, chickens were scarce and expensive, not reared commercially, and not available at the neighborhood grocery store or butcher shop. They were only available seasonally and not all year. It may seem difficult to believe, but your grandparents or great grandparents did not consume chicken in the same proportion as you do today.

The poultry industry is expected to exceed 425 billion USD by 2025, up from roughly 325 billion USD in 2022. Such astonishing figures could not have been achieved using sustainable farming practices. The research on white flesh (chicken meat) is still in its early stages, and only time will tell. After all, the chicken on your platter is not humble!

10. Similarly, with intensive exploitation, fish populations in seas and oceans are rapidly depleting. This has resulted in a fish farming spawning business in which fish are packed and bred in confined enclosures, leading to the fast spread of illnesses. According to some estimates, over 60-70% of all salmon is farmed.

After all, the unassuming salmon that is said to be incredibly nutritious and high in Omega-3 is not a salmon.

Chemicals, where antibiotics are freely employed, chemicals such as hydrogen peroxide are used to cure sea lice, they are fed pellets made of genetically changed soy and cornstarch, and they have the lowest Omega-3 fatty acid levels.

11. The meat on your plate may appear to be healthy and taste better, but it isn't and is riddled with chemicals.

And, unlike vegetables and fruits, the chemicals cannot be washed away. Modern farms forcibly feed animals soy and maize meal in order for them to gain weight quickly. Soy and Maize are grown using modern agricultural techniques we talked about earlier.

So, the chicken, fish, pig, lamb, and so on (any animal that is mass produced) are not as nutrient dense since swaths of forest land are cut to grow soy, while soy is grown utilizing current agricultural practices that I discussed previously. There is no way out of this vicious spiral. The solution is free range animals, but they are expensive and difficult to get.

Free-range animals and chickens, grass-fed animals (cow for dairy and beef, lamb, sheep, and so on), grains, vegetables, and fruits are your best chance.

Even if you have found a way out and can buy meat

from free-roaming animals/birds, you may not be getting your daily intake of micronutrients unless you eat animal organs.

You should think twice before eating muscle meat or any other bodily part because it may not meet your nutritional needs. The solution to the meat consumption dilemma is not simple.

Meat consumption is inextricably linked to our cultures, religious preferences, social fabric, festivals, holidays, and so on, and it is nearly difficult (but reasonable) to avoid meat.

What is also indisputable is that humans have not lived and flourished entirely on meat; for example, the Eskimo tribe has lived the most extreme carnivore diet, consuming just meat for nearly 10 months of the year; however, during spring, Eskimos devour grass, leaves, seeds, and fruits!

Although plant-based food consumption varies, humans have lived for thousands of years on an omnivorous diet.

Plant-based diets are not the holy grail either; if not balanced, they can contribute to nutritional deficiencies:

1. Vitamin B12- Studies ([89],[90]) have showed that vegetarians may be deficient in vitamin B. Vegans may connect to this because your doctor may have

recommended Vitamin B complex supplements; perhaps, vitamin B deficiency is to blame for your mouth ulcers.

Many vegetarian civilizations, however, have discovered a way around this by consuming dairy products (particularly yoghurt or curd), fermented food, and sprouts.

2. Iron absorption- Research[91] has shown that humans absorb iron more efficiently from animal sources (i.e., blood or red meat and not from white meat). Many studies have found that vegans do not get enough iron from their plant-based diet ([92],[93],[94]). According to one study[95], a vegetarian diet has adequate amounts of iron, but the same is not bioavailable for people to absorb.

As discussed in the last chapter, fermentation and germination boost iron bioavailability, which is one method vegetarians may compensate.

High fructose- Modern farming techniques, as well as the development of hybrids, have resulted in sweeter fruits with greater fructose levels than naturally grown fruits.

Any severe shift in the ancestrally adopted vegetarian diet or transition from an omnivore to an herbivore diet may cause zinc, protein, calcium, vitamin, and other important mineral deficit.

I understand what you're thinking. If I were you, I'd

have inquired, "Hey, what's the way out?" Well, there isn't a simple answer.

However, here are a few suggestions.

Blue zone-I'd like to mention a book called "the blue zones," published by Author Dan Buettner, about studies he and his colleagues conducted on regions around the world where people lived extremely long. They dubbed these areas "blue zones."

A highly recommended read, the book focuses on five regions around the world, including Sardinia in Italy, Icaria in Greece, Okinawa in Japan, Nicoya in Costa Rica, and Loma Linda in California, where they discovered an unusually high number of nonagenarians and centenarians, or people who live to their 90s and 100s while remaining healthy.

It was discovered that people in blue zones lived 12 more quality years than an average person in the United States.

Dan Buettner and his colleagues identified nine cohorts responsible for their longevity, one of which was their nutrition.

Residents in the blue zones primarily consumed whole plants. The word "whole" should be emphasised because people in these places did not have access to processed food and had to rely on unprocessed food that was locally accessible. They consume what they produce.

Their plant-based diet included:

• seasonal vegetables

• pulses

• whole grains

• locally grown nuts

This fully aligns with what Michael Pollan mentioned in his book and may vindicate Paul McCartney as well. However, people in blue zones ate meat as well; for example, inhabitants in Icaria, Sardinia, and Okinawa ate fish. For completeness, nutrition is merely one of several factors influencing their lifetime.

The point I'm trying to make is that eating a well-balanced diet is extremely important, and incorporating plants has advantages and avoiding meat is unnecessary as long as we supplement our diet with whole plant foods. If you eat primarily meat, it's time to make those slight changes and begin introducing plant-based foods into your diet.

2. Eat seasonally and locally- Food demographics have shifted dramatically during the last few decades. The world genuinely has no borders, and food flows at breakneck speed around the globe. No single cuisine predominated during your forefathers' time; their nutrition was heavily influenced by location, season,

and opportunity. Look at every cuisine around the world; it makes use of locally available plants, vegetables, and meat. Your grandmothers ate food that was grown locally (within 100 miles or 150 kilometers) and seasonally, which meant they ate food that grew during that season. They couldn't consume mangoes in the winter or during the rainy season!

Consuming seasonally and locally was inextricably intertwined. Our bodies were originally tuned in to the natural cycles around us, where we were accustomed to absorbing nutrition provided in seasonal foods. Farmers in my home state of India, for example, grow Hyacinth Beans in the winter. The seed is so localized that when grown locally and seasonally; it provides a distinct scent that enhances the flavor of our curries.

Plants are programmed to develop and multiply in specific seasons, and while modern agricultural techniques have given us access to the same food even during the off season, one question we should ask is whether it is genuinely nutritious? However, the concept of local and seasonal eating that I am referring to is not new; you already understood intuitively that seasonal food is tastier, has more flavor, and is also healthier.

We have a symbiotic relationship with plants, just as they do with nature. We are a part of the whole, sharing the same environment as plants and other living beings. The seasonal changes that affect plants, both directly and indirectly, affect our well-being. Our forefathers had developed adaptations that were in line with nature over many generations. Even today, many festivals and cultural events around the globe revolve around seasons and seasonal meals.

Ritucharya is a notion recommended by Ayurveda, one of the oldest ancient medicine and literature on holistic living. Ritu means season and charya means routine. Ritucharya refers to a change in lifestyle and food to cope with the physical and emotional effects of seasonal changes. As per Ayurveda, if the body cannot adjust to the environmental pressures, it leads to dosha (meaning that which creates troubles or errors), ayurvedic literature gives specific dietary advice based on the seasons.

The issue with reinforcing the concept of seasonal-local consumption is that there is very little research on this aspect because there are too many variables such as your ethnicity, where you live, your age, nutritional and energy needs, and tracking this on a large population and deriving tangible results from the research is perhaps a herculean task.

One reason the blue zone has a high longevity rate is because of its demographic isolation, and people had to consume what they grew, and as a result, they ate locally and seasonally. Compare that to food grown out of season and shipped hundreds of thousands of kilometers (or miles) to our supermarkets.

Another study worth mentioning is the Stanford University study [96] on Hazda hunter gatherers in Tanzenia, in which their gut microbiota was evaluated for seasonality. It was discovered that the Hazda diet swings with seasons, as does their gut microbiota, and that their gut microbiome changes drastically with seasonal dietary variations.

They discovered that particular microorganisms decrease and then rebound dramatically, depending on the season. The study vindicates that our bodies were organically programmed to ingest seasonal vegetables; now, compare this to what your forefathers ate.

Did they ever eat something that wasn't in season? They rarely travelled the distances that modern humans do; they were limited to a certain radius and ate items cultivated locally. Because our forefathers were not as resourceful as we are and had limited access to food, they had to ration and store grains for out-of-season consumption and consume grains/ pulses/ vegetables in sync with the seasons.

I would argue that even meat eating was seasonal; for example, there was and still is huge animal slaughter during particular festivals and events, and important occasions such as marriages were held during the season when food was plentiful.

We have already learned that gut microbiota and its diversity are vital for optimal wellbeing, and minor dietary changes considerably affected it, with many microorganisms being permanently lost if we are not attentive with our diet.

The golden rule is to never change the diet we followed during our formative years. We are moving away from seasonal and local consumption because of industrialization, mass transportation, and new creative preservation techniques such as refrigeration.

Yes, the agricultural revolution provided us with dependability and a year-round access to food, it also resulted in mono crop dependency, with many societies becoming dependent on single staple crops such as rice, wheat, potatoes, and so on, reducing diversity and narrowing diets. According to research [97], contemporary [98]agriculture and reliance on single crops as an energy source are generating health problems, with nutritional inadequacies potentially leading to diseases.

It is time to eat produce at the farmers' market rather than the supermarket!

3. Watch the meat- Although eating meat is not necessarily harmful, it is best to do so in moderation. Try incorporating organ meat into your diet while avoiding processed meat. In addition, consume free range local meat and avoid farm bred meat.

4. Diversity-We already know this and have heard it in

various forms. Consuming various foods and including variation is one hallmark of balanced nutrition. People in the blue zone intuitively understood this, and their food was varied. Even now, there is a significant variation between the diets of rural and urban populations.

I've already mentioned how a diversified gut flora is an indicator of health and energy. Many studies[99] have showed that a healthy microbiome depends on a diverse diet.

The oxygen we breathe is paradoxical. It allows us to exist while also being a lethal killer, since it burns us from within, causing oxidative damage. Simply put, oxidative damage is the cost of breathing oxygen. Oxygen is what we need to survive. We take in clean air (of which oxygen is one component) and expel carbon dioxide. We ingest carbs, lipids, and protein (carbon and hydrogen chains) for energy, and our body mixes the carbon in carbohydrates with oxygen from clean air to expel carbon dioxide.

Oxidative stress is a natural occurrence and the cost of breathing, oxidative stress produces free radicals, as scientists refer to them. Understanding free radicals requires some knowledge of chemistry though. However, simplistically; unchecked free radicals, amongst others are responsible for host of health concerns including ageing and range of diseases. Oxidative stress causes inflammation in the body every day, minute by minute. Over millions of years, our bodies have eliminated free radicals.

Oxidative stress is exacerbated by nutrition (sugar and ultra-processed foods), environment (such as pollution), lifestyle (sedentary lifestyle), and other factors.

Humans have shared a symbiotic relationship with plants where they have been used for anti-inflammation and anti-oxidant capabilities for millions of years. Plants, like us, experience oxidative stress, as plants release oxygen as part of photosynthesis.

Plants manufacture phytochemical to protect themselves from oxidative damage; for clarity, phytochemical give plants their hues and effervescence (diverse colors). Plants, for example, produce Vitamin C, which has anti-oxidant qualities. Anti-oxidants basically neutralise the negative effects of free radicals and restore balance to the body. Fruits, vegetables, and pulses are high in phytochemical, which function as anti-inflammatory and antioxidants.

To reap the most advantages, we should load our plates with colorful phytochemicals every day, consuming a range of fruits, vegetables, cereals, and pulses as part of a daily balanced diet.

Dooms diet- Every diet will fail. Diet will not benefit you and may cause irreversible damage. Remember that the food you and your ancestors ate was the healthiest, and there is no reason to change it unless your doctor advises you otherwise.

Chapter 6
The body—made to move

Chapter 6 - The body: made to move

Let's begin with the obvious, physical activity is beneficial to our health. We already know that physical activity reduces the risk of mortality, cardiovascular disease, hypertension, type 2 diabetes, many types of cancer, dementia Alzheimer's, anxiety, depression, sleep issues, bone loss, and bone breaking, to mention a few.

Contrary to common assumption, physical activity is not a way to reduce weight; rather, it is a way to stay healthy. We previously learned in the myth chapter that losing weight with calorie restriction and exercise is a double-edged sword. The Problem is that we have been looking for the incorrect strategy. We want to lose weight before getting healthy. I advocate getting healthy and losing weight in the process. Losing weight with the former approach is easier, whereas losing weight with the latter is more difficult.

Exercise has never helped people maintain their weight loss. Weight reduction through exercise is moderate, according to a large body of study.[100] The study found that disrupting appetite hormones for an extended period inclined participant to gain weight.

Another study revealed[101] that weight loss generated considerable compensatory reductions in energy consumption that counteracted with long-term weight loss (meaning people consumed more energy on days of exercise). Changes caused by rapid weight loss include increased appetite (insatiable to where people binge), lack of energy, emotional instability, and so on.

Unfortunately, there is an information overload in which healthcare experts, the media, and the public believe that exercise (often intense exercise) can cause weight loss.

People who have tried and failed will tell you from personal experience that they have lost weight and gained it all back, which creates a negative feedback loop and conditioning in which people lose confidence and eventually despise physical activity, leading them to forsake exercise.

The issue is that we have been looking for a solution at the wrong door. The secret to weight loss is not exercise; it is instilling a healthy lifestyle; with patience and effort, you will find the sweet spot!

It is also important to note that our body is designed to move; let me explain with a few examples:

Although our surrounds and the environment in which we live have transformed over the last few centuries, we continue to inhabit the same bodies that we developed over 200,000 years ago. Yes, we live in the same body that 200,000 years ago ran, walked, leaped, climbed, crawled, and foraged (just look at children in the park).

We are guilty of prolonged sitting even when compared to our parents or grandparents, and we have re-engineered our environment to suit sedentary lifestyles, such as having machines do our daily chores, having a couch at home, and spending an increasing amount of time sitting on chairs or inside a car.

If 200,000 years is a long period, the re-engineering that I alluded to is a relatively recent phenomenon that has resulted in people sitting more and moving less (as early as a few decades). Movement was critical to human evolution and the survival of our species.

People in blue zones, for example, hardly engaged in exercise because locomotion was embedded in their lifestyle, where people moved around instead of using transportation, they lived in terrains, they used to do their own chores even in the late stages of their lives, people from a few regions sat on the floor where the act of sitting and getting up multiple times served as *micro exercises*.

Isn't it self-evident that these are micro-exercises?

1. The benefits of repeating micro workouts throughout the day are enormous.

2. The human leg, [102]for example, is built for running. Humans' tiny toes and long legs make long distance running simpler.

3. Other associated adaptations for movement and running include bigger[103] gluteus muscles (buttocks), a small waist, neck thoracic flexibility, and increased flexibility of vestibular and ocular reflexes. Pigs, for example, are not built to run, and they are clumsy runners. If you look at YouTube footage of running pigs, you observe that the pig's head wobbles excessively when running. As a result, they are clumsy and prone to falling. In comparison, humans have visual, mental, and bodily adaptations that are specifically developed for running.

4. Our metabolism, i.e., our ability to regulate our internal temperature, is intended for endurance and long-term movements.

5. Physical activity has a variety of beneficial effects on the human brain, one of which is neurogenesis (meaning production of new neurons). Aerobic exercise boosts the anterior hippocampus, or human memory region ([104] and [105]). According [106] to one study, exercising improves[107] memory.

6. There is a direct relationship between increasing physical activity and the expansion of the hippocampus and several other brain regions.

The advantages, relationships, and biological adaptations are clear, and much of it you already know, yet we find it tough to wake up every day and get moving.

Why, one could ask? For much of human history, people have engaged in physical activities for **a**. survival (hunting, collecting, fleeing predators, etc.) or **b**. recreation (dancing, competitive sport etc.,) **c**. There may be some people who are inherently athletic.

Our grandparents did not have access to the many equipment that we use today for tasks; they had to do it all by themselves; they did not have easy access to resources as modern humans do, and they had to walk medium to short distances to get food.

They also lacked the transportation that the current generation does, which resulted in micro-exercises throughout the day. Being sedentary is an acquired habit rather than an underlying human trait.

We were very active throughout our youth and teens. Inactivity creeps in throughout our undergraduate years and is exacerbated when we begin a desk job. The Reasons may be many, but we have unconsciously conditioned ourselves to inactivity.

Perhaps one reason we were otherwise active was that the physical activity was recreational and competitive, with both characteristics driving the drive to move. As time passes, both recreation and competition, as well as motivation, take a second seat.

Even so-called athletic students in high school and college become less active and more sedentary. We find it difficult to inspire ourselves to move unless it is for fun or as part of a competition.

You may have witnessed this at your team offsite or team get together where your colleagues break stereotypes and engage in intensive physical activity as part of team sports and appear to thrive on it.

The proclivity for inactivity may be related to a change in environment (from an active and frolic lifestyle to one where education/grades matter, resulting in endless hours of sitting and preparation), moving into a new job, work stress, getting married, having children, and so on, but the result is inactivity.

Physical exercise is easy to avoid; we can't live without eating every day, but we can live with very little physical activity. When they are not hunting or gathering, the Hazda spends a lot of time sitting. However, it was discovered that dancing (high intensity dance) is engrained in their culture, with young and old alike taking part in dance as part of ceremonies and enjoyment.

The point I'm trying to make here is that physical exercise is not second nature to humans; historically, we've engaged in a physical activity for survival (i.e., hunting or gathering), recreation (such as dancing or playing entertaining games with friends), or vocational reasons (such as athletes).

To be sure, each person's problem and solution are unique, but the benefits of physical activity are unquestionably enormous, spanning both physiological and psychological benefits. Given this, how can one include physical activity into one's everyday routine?

Here are a few easy recommendations:

Chore is the new exercise - Do housework at least once a week, gradually increasing the frequency. The act of cleaning vessels raises the heart rate. Cleaning the floor work your shoulder, leg, and back muscles, acting as micro-exercises.

Walk while you talk - People who work at a desk grumble about unending meetings and phone calls. Why not use the meetings to perform micro-exercises? Whereas you can walk while talking or listening, not all calls will require you to sit in front of a screen.

Stand while you work-Instead of sitting on a chair all day, use a standing work bench. Breaking the sitting cycle provides metabolic benefits. When you stand, your body needs to work against gravity, which engages specific muscles that are not engaged when you sit.

Sit less and walk more-Walk/ cycle to the nearest grocery store instead of driving. Walk to the bus stop, and if you take a cab, select a pickup spot that is 5-10 minutes away from your typical pickup location. Park your car somewhere far away and walk to the appointed location.

Climb rather than stand-Use the stairs instead of escalators or lifts. Climbing uses your muscles, strengthens them, and provides fantastic cardio.

Take a mini break-While work might be stressful and taking a break may seem difficult, it is always beneficial to take a small 10-15-minute break and go for a little walk; it is refreshing and a great stress buster.

Find a buddy-taking part in play time on weekends or in your leisure time. As previously said, we appear to fare better when we engage in physical activity for fun or as part of a competition.

Shake a leg! Dancing raises your heart rate and works several muscles. Dancing is both good for your health and enjoyable.

Plant a garden - Digging, planting, weeding, and picking are all micro-exercises, plus gardening offers a lot of psychological advantages.

Nature stroll-Get out of the house and go for a walk in your neighborhood park. This also has significant psychological benefits.

Play with your child-Children are a bundle of energy, and even 30 minutes of play with them will help you reap enormous benefits.

Chores, standing while you talk, and going the additional mile may all appear undesirable on the surface. They are uninteresting because we see no purpose in them and our mind trivialises the benefits.

People who have children understand that getting children to do chores or run/walk is easier said than done. They may perform it a few times before becoming bored. But we aren't any different.

However, if you transform the unappealing action into a game and give it a purpose, the child in you will love it and may continue to do so until it becomes a habit.

Similarly, give your chore/activity significance and purpose, instill passion, and have a goal in mind. It's like your boss assigning you a task with a deadline. A motivated and enthusiastic mind will find joy and thrive on little things.

Chapter 7

Fasting, the supreme medicine!

Chapter 7 - Fasting, the supreme medicine!

Let me guess. This chapter should come as no surprise, and you may think, yet another guy writing about fasting! Yes, you've probably heard and read a lot about fasting and its benefits. "Intermittent fasting" is the latest buzzword in town; your friends seem to practice it, and you may have tried it yourself. But the question is how many of them (including you) have kept it going?

Intermittent fasting is currently popular all over the world. I've always wondered why they use the prefix (intermittent) before fasting. Fasting, by definition, implies abstaining from food for a set period (i.e., intermittently) while not starving!

The mind is an intriguing machine. It will not commit unless it is completely convinced; for it to commit, it needs a purpose, a passion, and a belief. The problem is that what worked for someone else is not a strong enough motivation for the mind to commit, and the urge fades quickly, and people return to their old behaviors. Societal pressure and constant feedback exacerbates the problem. You seem to encounter more sceptics and detractors than true encouragers and motivators.

My fasting path has been fraught with difficulties, and my family was originally unsupportive. They were both terrified and doubtful. Even now, my in-laws and my mother think I've gone insane! My methods were validated when my wife experienced actual benefits and followed in my footsteps, embarking on this adventure with me for the past five years. For the past six years, I have practiced fasting and its ways (one year before my wife joined me).

It was a life-altering and eye-opening experience. The most apparent effect of fasting is weight loss; however, fasting has many other benefits that are unique to each individual. Fasting is a beautiful experience. When you embark on a fasting journey, your body and mind become addicted to it (healthily), and you are soon married to fasting for life. It also makes you question how and why you were eating so much during the day.

"Langhanam Parama Aushadam," states a poem in Indian Ayurvedic literature, literally meaning "Fasting is the supreme treatment." Pratyahar, which means abstention from food, is also mentioned in Ayurveda. Fasting is considered a therapeutic cure during the commencement of fever in Ayurvedic literature as jvardau langhanam proctam, which translates to "at the onset of fever, fast". In his literary works, Indian Saint Vagbhatt Rishi lists the benefits of fasting as "disappearance of severe faults in the body, strengthening of the digestive fire, weight reduction, enhanced energy and vitality, removal of toxins, actual hunger and thirst, and the desire to eat." People share this belief all throughout the world; Hippocrates, for example, stated that "to eat when you are sick is to feed your ailment." Hippocrates is regarded as the father of modern medicine, and he advocated fasting as the first line of defence and medication. "A little fasting can truly do more for the average sick man than the best medicines and the best doctors," Mark Twain once said. The famed American scientist Benjamin Franklin advised, "The best of all remedies is rest and fasting." My experience resonates with these statements.

Fasting has been my cold and fever treatment for many years; my recovery rate is faster, and my symptoms last less time. The only drug I've taken (sparingly) is paracetamol for fever, and only at my family's request. There is additional evidence that the body engages in self-induced food limitation to sustain fever and other protective processes.

Through millions of years of evolution, our bodies have naturally developed mechanisms to reducing weight and keeping healthy through the natural process of fasting, and we have naturally calibrated our bodies to burn fat during times of food shortage and build fat during times of food abundance. Although this appears to be straightforward, we find it difficult to believe and are often afraid to even try.

Fasting was observed by various ancient societies, including Egypt, Syria, Scythia, Greece, Babylon, Persia, Nineveh, Palestine, Rome, and China, as well as the Druids, Celts, Scandinavians, Indians of North America, and Aztecs and Incas of South America.

Fasting was a way of life for hunter gatherers who were subject to the whims of nature and had to subsist with meagre food for many days before bingeing when food was abundant.

Despite the agricultural revolution's ease of access to food, approximately 10% of the world's population still goes to bed hungry. Fasting as a survival and growth technique has existed from the beginning of life on Earth (nearly 4 billion years). Many organisms, including animals and humans, had learned to live during times of drought and food scarcity.

During times of food scarcity, many organisms and animals fall into hibernation mode to conserve energy. Many animals, including the polar bear, hibernate during the winter, subsisting on stored body fat.

We are no different because we share the same ancestors.

Do you recall bingeing when you had a fever? On days when we aren't feeling well, we intuitively lower our food intake and skip meals. Fasting is an intuitive response that comes naturally to humans. Unless someone reminds us, we take these details for granted.

With the agricultural revolution and easy availability to food, our forefathers devised inventive and spiritual methods of self-control, such as fasting, as many cultures and faiths explicitly promote fasting as a way of life. Fasting has been an element of religious and health traditions throughout history. Fasting was practised by most societies as recently as 50 years ago, but it has faded with the agricultural/industrial revolution.

Even now, many orthodox and religious people fast as a traditional practise. A few notable faiths that promote dietary abstinence are (in no particular order):

Muslims practise fasting throughout the holy month of Ramadan, which lasts between 29 and 30 days. During this month, Muslims refrain from eating or drinking during the day.

Hinduism-Hindus fast for religious and penitential reasons. We mainly observe fasting during the many festivals, when people refrain from eating and only eat after the food has been donated to the deity. They also practised fasting as part of the lunar cycle (Ekadashi and Purnima), during which no food is ingested for 16-48 hours.

Fasting comes in a variety of forms and flavors, including ektana (one cooked meal each day) and dharna-parna (food one day and fast the next day). Certain religious sects consume and abstain from certain foods during certain months (also known as Chaturmas), and most of the festivals take place during this time.

Hindus observed fasting as self-denial to please their deity or as penance to wash away one's sins. Many societies used to fast as a kind of self-discipline, with monks and priests abstaining from meals for extended periods of time to refine self-control and regulate the mind and body. Different sects and subsects of Hinduism observe fasting at different periods and frequencies.

Christianity –Lent is the season where Christians, (Catholics), give up a certain food or practice fasting. Within Christianity, different sects follow fasting at different times and frequency.

Other cultures- Fasting is practised in certain societies for non-religious reasons. In Japan, for example, skipping breakfast is common. In Switzerland, a day is set aside for fasting, which is usually a public holiday.

Blue zones - People in Ikaria's blue zone region frequently fast for over 150 days for religious reasons.

"OK, this is useful to know," you would think. Is there any tangible advantage"? Let's delve a little deeper. Fasting has recently gained a negative connotation, with fasting being equated with famine. Have you ever wondered why the meal you have a first thing in the morning is referred to as breakfast? It shows that you are *break*ing a *fast*. We normally have dinner at 8 p.m. and breakfast at 8 a.m. the following morning. This means we've been fasting for 12 hours. It does not imply that you have been starving for 12 hours.

There have been days when we have delayed or entirely skipped breakfast (current research shows that almost one-third of Chinese skip breakfast because of a lack of time); this would imply that we have previously practised fasting in either case, but not consciously or as a lifestyle change. Let's dispel some myths and clear up some misunderstandings.

For a long time, we have been taught that breakfast is the most important meal of the day, but breakfast (an English word) does not have an equivalent word in many countries or cultures. Our current eating pattern of three meals a day plus snacks with fruit juice or coffee/tea in between has no scientific basis. People ate one or two meals every day during most human history. For example, I come from a priestly family in India, and our forefathers never ate breakfast, instead ate lunch between 12 and 1 p.m.

Even now, orthodox members of my community do not have breakfast; in fact, there is no such thing as breakfast in my culture. Breakfast was non-existent throughout the mediaeval times in Britain and Europe, where the term originated (around 100 to 500 years ago).

Breakfast may have been developed as a survival mechanism for youngsters, the elderly, the sick, and working-class members of society because physical labor was difficult and the energy requirements were quite high as compared to aristocrats and white collared working-class members (i.e., people with desk jobs in the modern age).

The contemporary obsession with three meals a day with snacks in between could be attributed to our ability to grow and store food, which resulted in a shift in our eating habits. Convenience is the mother of creativity, and humans began designing foods to meet our needs for many three meals each day. We created rituals and cultures around it; it is difficult to comprehend that two meals were once the norm in the 18th and 19th century. We still believe and are afraid when someone suggests skipping a meal, no matter how hard we try!

I know I am entering a risky area, as breakfast is a sensitive subject with many layers of culture, everyday practice, emotions, and history wrapped around it. Dissecting each of these angles is time-consuming and may require its own book.

However, we may look at the adaptations that our bodies have built over millions of years of evolution to gain insight into the importance or otherwise of breakfast. If you have or have had a diabetic in your household, you know already that their blood test is divided into two phases: before and after meals.

Diabetes patients, interestingly, have higher blood glucose levels in their fasting blood sample. Have you ever wondered why a glucose blood test is performed before a meal and why they have high glucose levels?

In the realm of diabetics, this is known as the Dawn Phenomenon, in which the blood glucose level rises dramatically without insulin really counteracting it (remember insulin is not released in type 1 diabetics and people with type 2 diabetes either do not produce enough insulin or if at all the insulin is produced, it is unable to perform its function in the body (insulin resistance)).

The question is, how does our body release glucose into the bloodstream before we eat our first meal? Early in the morning (typically around 3 a.m.), your body is attempting to prepare itself for the day ahead and wants to give you an advantage because ancient humans were supposed to venture outside to hunt or gather food, and the body releases growth hormone, cortisol, and glucagon, stimulating the liver to produce and release glucose into the bloodstream. This offers your body a push and an energy boost to get you ready for the day ahead. Your body is already in high gear, anticipating the day ahead. Food is actually at the bottom of the list.

If you're asking if this just happens among diabetics, the answer is no. This is a natural phenomenon in humans, and our bodies repeat it every day in the morning; the spike in glucose causes cells in the pancreas to generate insulin to help maintain blood sugar levels balanced, and the result? Energy - where your organs and cells get a burst of energy in the morning. What would happen if you ate first thing in the morning to fuel an already energised body? The answer is simple—weight gain!

It is vital to notice that the body does not provide you with a burst of energy in the morning; rather, the process is sluggish and energy is released gradually over many hours. But you're probably wondering why you're hungry in the morning. Morning hunger is a conditioned behavior from childhood in which we are regularly taught to have breakfast early in the morning and our bodies become accustomed to this routine.

"Eat breakfast like a king, lunch like a prince, and dinner like a pauper" my teacher used to say when I was a kid. The question is, how accurate is this, and can you truly eat like a pauper and survive?

According to studies[108], the portion size of lunch and dinner remains constant regardless of the quantity of breakfast, so you may have breakfast like a king but that doesn't mean you can sustain having dinner like a pauper, your body and mind will eventually force you to have proper dinner (and not pauper dinner!), and the result? Breakfast overeating causes weight gain.

Ironically, eating like a king may cause an obese monarch! A study found that eating breakfast has little effect on weight gain or loss when other factors are considered (such as physical activity, a low-calorie diet, and so on). The study recommends a low-calorie diet combined with physical activity, but cautions that there are tangible benefits if only diet and physical activity are maintained.

Breakfast alone will not make a person fat or skinny; it is a mix of factors such as what we eat during breakfast (sugar and UPF), our predispositions, age (the calorie requirement for children and adolescents are greater when compared with adults), the timing of dinner, and so on. It is therefore misleading to claim that children and teenagers should have two meals a day as their calorie requirement is different to adults.

However, there has never been a persuasive study that has recommended or emphasised the importance of breakfast, and I have not come across any study that claims that skipping breakfast is damaging to human health (few observational research papers say breakfast is important).

According to the findings of a 2019 evaluation[109] of 13 randomized control trials, the addition of breakfast may not be a beneficial weight loss approach. Breakfast, contrary to popular opinion, is not the most important meal of the day, and skipping breakfast is not hazardous.

Breakfast abstinence is a simple and risk-free way to lose weight. Although there is no substantive evidence linking breakfast to weight gain, there is evidence that skipping breakfast results in weight loss, and there are no studies that claim skipping breakfast makes you fat!

If you're still not persuaded, try listening to your body, eat breakfast or any meal only when you're hungry, and your body may tell you the answer. And if you become hungry, avoid eating the chocolate, cookie, slice of bread, or other UPF. Instead, have some fruit or a salad.

My quest began with similar cynicism; the beginnings were modest, with me delaying breakfast by 30 minutes and increasing by 30 minutes every week. My body adjusted gradually, and after a few months, I was in the habit of having brunch at 12:30 p.m. Nowadays, I'm not sure why I had breakfast at all! Let's debunk few popular misconceptions around fasting.

Eating regularly - There is a prevalent misconception that eating six small meals a day is preferable to two large meals, and that eating frequently helps you lose weight. I debunked this fallacy in the insulin chapter. Eating regularly keeps your pancreas on high alert, where it will continue to pump insulin, and we all know that insulin is a double-edged sword because it slows fat burn.

Fasting is detrimental for your health-While fasting has many health benefits, no study has ever found that it is bad for your health.

Fasting does not make you overeat in order to compensate. I know from personal experience it is nearly impossible to gorge and binge on food after fasting. With a smaller portion, the body feels satisfied. I've never overeaten after a fast. Yet, if you tend to overeat in the feeding window, it will offset the benefits you have derived.

Okay, fasting has been practised throughout human history. We have developed the ability to function for extended periods of time without eating. Fasting is a more natural adaptation than eating several meals throughout the day. The question requires an answer: how can fasting benefit me, and are there any drawbacks?

In the following paragraphs, we will learn about the benefits and drawbacks of fasting so that you may make an informed decision and make a lifestyle change.

Weight Loss: Fasting is an effective weight loss method. Our basic sources of energy are via the food we eat (such as carbohydrate) or stored energy (such as glycogen stored by the liver, fat stored in tissues, or protein stored in muscles). The obvious and sole reason our bodies store energy is to use it when food is scarce. Our bodies have developed mechanisms for converting stored energy (fat) to useful energy.

At the most basic level, the body goes through two phases: feeding and fasting (also known as the metabolic switch). In the insulin chapter, we learned about the feeding[110] and fasting phases. But, for the sake of clarity, let me repeat:

Fasting begins roughly 8 hours after the last meal, when the glucose from the feeding phase is totally exhausted and the liver utilizes stored glycogen for energy requirements via a cascade of metabolic events. This happens about 12 hours after the last meal.

In the insulin chapter, we explored how the liver converts stored glycogen to glucose, causing the pancreas to release insulin to offset the glucose release.

Insulin levels then decline, as does glycogen storage. Your liver should now seek alternative energy sources. When glucose levels fall, the pancreas directs the liver to create new glucose, which the liver does by using amino acids and glycerol.

As fasting continues, the body uses stored fat as a potential energy source. Fat is broken down and released into the bloodstream, where it is converted by the liver into a more useful energy form known as ketones. Ketones (an alternate energy source for cells to glucose) are how energy is delivered to your cells and brain while fasting. This procedure is also called as ketosis.

Each stage lasts from 8 hours after a meal to 72 hours, with the actual rate and timing varying by individual. According to research[111], the body can enter ketosis as soon as 12 hours after eating.

We are well aware of the damage that unabated insulin causes in our bodies. One important principle to remember is that fat burning ceases with insulin release. Although these adaptations serve a purpose, excess insulin and insulin resistance are the leading causes of obesity and, as a result, the key to weight management.

However, insulin is not the sole reason fasting and weight loss are linked. Weight control is the product of a complicated interplay of several factors. Here are some important reasons:

Insulin resistance and sensitivity-We already know that insulin resistance is one reason we can't lose weight and why weight rebounds after calorie restriction and exercise.

Calorie restriction (i.e., diet) combined with exercise does not treat the underlying problem (i.e., insulin resistance) ([112]) as any weight lost is quickly replaced, and we are back to square one.

Insulin resistance occurs when your cells cannot respond to insulin generated by the pancreas and so become resistant and, as a result, less sensitive (insulin sensitivity). Humans who are at their ideal weight are insulin sensitive where the cells react to insulin, so the body absorbs glucose as quickly as insulin is released, neutralizing both insulin and glucose. In a healthy person, this conforming adaption occurs naturally. Obese or overweight people are insulin resistant and insensitive, leading to weight increase and a vicious cycle.

Where calorie restriction fails, fasting succeeds. Fasting increases the sensitivity of cells to insulin, resulting in a decline in blood sugar and insulin levels. Lower insulin levels make stored fat more accessible to the liver, leading in fat loss. When compared to calorie restriction regimens, one study[113] found that intermittent fasting is an efficient strategy to lose weight.

Appetite and Metabolism-Another advantage of fasting is that it regulates appetite by decreasing[114] the hungry hormone (ghrelin) and increasing the feeling of fullness, resulting in less food cravings ([115], [116]). These components work together to inhibit overeating, making it harder to gorge or binge after fasting. Fasting causes the adrenal glands and neurons to release a hormone called norepinephrine, commonly known as adrenaline, which serves as a hormone and neurotransmitter (a substance that sends signals between nerve cells). Norepinephrine is a fat-burning hormone that mobilizes the brain and body for action. Fasting increases the amount of this fat-burning hormone produced and released. The primary cause of the higher metabolic rate is norepinephrine. A faster metabolism shows that the fasting body is in fat-burning mode.

Fasting for brief durations, contrary to popular opinion, does not make you sleepy (i.e., slower metabolism); the body is really attentive and active; it is burning fat and generating hormones (Norepinephrine) that give you more energy to go out and seek food.

This makes sense because hunter gatherers would need energy to go out and hunt or scavenge. A rising amount of research[117] shows that ketones, rather than glucose, are the preferred energy source for the body. Through the precise orchestration of hormones, fasting assaults body fat from many perspectives. It raises metabolic rate (burns more calories) and decreases food intake (reduces calories in).

Fasting for 16-18 hours per day will cause fat loss and weight loss. Many researches have connected weight loss to time restricted eating and feeding ([118], [119], [120],

[121]). In fact, there is significant weight reduction [122] (3%-8%) in the first days of fasting (3 to 24 weeks); this is quite astounding given the short timeframe. There is a significant reduction in waist circumference (4%-7%) during the initial phase.

Human Growth Hormone (HGH or growth hormone)-Growth Hormone is produced by the pituitary gland. In children and teenagers, this hormone regulates growth. It aids in regulating body composition, fluids, muscle and bone growth, fat metabolism, healing from injury and disease, and maybe heart function in adults.

Growth hormone deficiency[123] can cause decreased muscle mass, increased fat mass, with excess fat accumulating around the waist and predominantly visceral (meaning around the abdominal internal organs); this is also associated with a lower life expectancy and an increased risk of cardiovascular (heart) disease; low HGH results in a lower quality of life, an increased risk of disease, and an increased risk of weight gain. It is also worth noting that optimal HGH[124] is a vital factor in persons who desire to lose weight.

Interestingly, research has revealed that increased body fat has a direct effect on HGH levels[125], which are lower in obese persons, particularly males, and that lowering belly fat miraculously[126] returns HGH levels to normal range.

People who have more stored fat appear to have lower HGH levels.

Increased insulin levels appear to have a negative effect on HGH production, as higher insulin interrupts HGH production [127]. Fasting has a significant impact on HGH modulation.

According to studies [128,129] there is a surge in growth hormone during fasting, with HGH doubling/tripling during the first few days of fasting. Fasting can have a knock-on effect on HGH levels.

Fasting fat burn promotes HGH production while also lowering insulin levels; as a result, HGH levels are driven and surge during fasting. Aside from weight loss, a few notable direct and indirect benefits are:

1. Autophagy-As previously said, organisms intuitively fast during disease and then resume eating when they recover.

When starved, cells in the body enter autophagy (meaning "eat oneself") mode, in which deteriorated, damaged, and old cell parts, as well as microbes (bacterial and viruses), are detected and recycled into their components to supply energy and building blocks for cell renewal. The body eliminates old/damaged cells, poisons, and pathogens while generating newer, healthier cells.

Autophagy is the body's natural housekeeping function that keeps cells healthy ([130]). This is a key function, yet the precise procedure was unknown until Japanese cell biologist Yoshinori Houma identified autophagy genes while working on yeast cells. He was awarded the Nobel Prize in Physiology or Medicine in 2016 for uncovering the principles of autophagy.

Fasting for 12 to 24 hours has been discovered to start autophagy, which is one reason fasting is related with increased lifespan (anti-ageing). Fasting-induced autophagy has been shown in studies to provide a variety of health effects.

Autophagy is the body's mechanism of rewinding time, in which old, damaged cells are eliminated and replaced with new cells ([131]). Fasting, through autophagy, literally makes you biologically younger. Although research in this area is still in its early stages, fasting-induced autophagy may be a viable cancer treatment ([132]). Fasting-induced autophagy has anti-inflammatory benefits ([133]).

2. Makes your life easier-

Yes, those who fast will find it easier to manage their lives since they will have one less meal to prepare or one day where they will not have to cook or eat out. It also frees up a lot of time that would otherwise be spent cooking or going out to eat.

We invariably have one meal in our three meals a day mindlessly where you don't even realise what you just ate, three meals a day together with snacks is mechanical; skipping a meal will allow you to love your meals. This is also much easier than calorie counting because you don't need special foods and you can stop calculating calories; all you need to do is eat healthy and whole foods during feasting times and avoid ultra-processed foods and sugar.

You may already be eating in this manner regularly, with an early dinner and a late morning breakfast. All it takes is a little tweaking and a bit of tuning to your current diet.

You will surely get enormous benefits by changing your current diet and eating healthy during the eating window. So, you like the concept, you want to try, but you're not sure where to begin.

Here's the solution:

You can find a ton of literature on various fasting methods and how to actually implement them on the internet; I do not plan to regurgitate what is already accessible. However, I could describe the approaches that I have used and advised to my students. There is no hard and fast rule or one-size-fits-all solution. You should start small, try a few approaches, and then settle on one, as I did.

Each body will react differently, therefore, it is critical that you listen to your body and do not follow the rules. Don't get drawn into it, and don't keep it too close to your heart, because it might lead to painful heartbreak if things don't go as planned. Remember, this is a lifelong shift, not a quick fix.

I've also seen that while individuals are eager to get on the fasting bandwagon, most cannot do so since they must overcome certain mental hurdles in order to succeed with the fasting methods. In my personal experience, some self-defeating thought patterns should be avoided, such as; Negative self-talk and peer talk like - Am I doing it right? Why am I exhausted? Will fasting cause me to become malnourished? Did I get a fever from fasting? Why am I feeling so frail? What you're doing is improper; you've grown frail, he never listens to us, and so forth.

I had to deal with internal, family, and societal pressure, where self-talk became overpowering and quickly devolved into self-defeating conversations.

These thoughts are strong and persistent, and they are impossible to ignore. However, the remedy is not simple. My way out was to stay focused on the bigger picture and the process rather than getting bogged down in details. All is said and done. If our mind can be self-critical, it can also think favorably, and the option is ours.

Yes, it can be lonely; I was unwaveringly optimistic about the journey. The key is to identify like-minded people and a mentor who can guide you through the early stages. Please contact me if you require any advice or believe you are moving in the wrong direction.

Internal convictions and unwritten rules- The most crucial meal of the day is breakfast. I can't say no to food when it's provided to me, etc. The irony of internal beliefs and unwritten norms is that the abnormalities can be explained logically or scientifically. The only way out of this is to seek knowledge and break free from your unfounded ideas. There may be times when you find it difficult to stick to your methods because of societal pressure (an occasion, or holiday, for example); honestly, it should be okay to break the pattern once in a while in order to conform to society or unique situation; don't be hard on yourself and always remember, you are in it for the long haul and one or few days of non-adherence is okay in the interest of social conformity.

Now that we've covered the mental aspect, let's have a look at some of the most popular fasting methods, and I'll also tell you what has worked best for me.

There is no set length for fasting, and there is no measurement. Fasting can last anywhere from 12 hours to several months. Choose the optimal fasting window that you are comfortable. Pay attention to your body. However, here are a few well-known (and proven and true) fasting techniques:

16:8 - You eat dinner early in the evening (usually before 8 p.m.), skip breakfast the next morning, and eat an early lunch the next day (typically at 12 pm).

You will end up with an 8-hour eating window where you can consume normal stuff. This is the most straightforward method to implement and maintain. Intuitively, this will quickly become a lifestyle change.

The nicest part about 16:8 is that you are bound to miss lunch at 12 on a few days (perhaps have lunch at 1 pm), which means you are doing 18:8 on some days and 16:8 on others. This has been the most effective method for me over the last six years.

If you find it impossible to forgo breakfast (say, at 9 a.m.), have an early dinner (before 5 pm). The only drawback to this method is that you may wake up hungry in the middle of the night. As I already stated, pay attention to your body. If your body accepts this approach, go ahead.

20:4—This extends the 16:8 paradigm, in which you feed for four hours and fast for twenty. This requires some training and I would not recommend it for novices. While you can achieve 16:8 every day, 20:4 may be challenging to maintain daily because of your mind creating phantom hunger and constantly reminding you. I struggled with this and returned to

16:8.

One meal a day (OMAD)-As the name implies, we only eat one meal per day, usually dinner. You eat dinner at 8 p.m. on day one and again at 8 p.m. on day two. On day 3, you will eat lunch at 12 p.m.

On day 2, the meal is often light, not filling the stomach, and free of UPF and sugar. This means you've only had two meals in a 40 hours window, and you've avoided UPF and sugar during that time. Personally, this has worked brilliantly for me. Six days a week, I do 16:8 and once a week; I do OMAD. The problem with OMAD is that if you are around food (for example, your house where your family is eating three meals a day, or an office party where they cut a birthday cake); it becomes painfully difficult to resist eating. As a result, I don't practice OMAD at home unless my wife and I practice together.

5:2-This is the most difficult to accomplish; it takes determination and practice. For the first five days, you eat three meals a day and fast for two. A few of my friends and students have even tried a 5:2 and 16:8 hybrid, in which you only eat two meals per day for five days instead of three. There are a handful that advocate 500 calories on fasting days. Personally, I do not suggest this strategy because it does not promote habit building. 500 calories on fasting days falls into the realm of calorie counting and restriction, which I neither appreciate nor encourage. Instead, if you have the ability and willpower, I advocate a 48-hour continuous fast. However, 16:8 and OMAD are equally effective.

Important: If you have any underlying medical conditions, please get advice from your doctor.

To be honest, it makes little difference whichever technique of fasting you use as long as you do one of them. Before you begin, there are a few things you should consider:

Don't eat sugar in the fasting window. The issue with sugar is that it causes the pancreas to generate insulin, which immediately stops fat burning.

Drink plenty of water, but don't go overboard with it. Remember, your body knows best, and it requires hydration during fasting. Dehydration is a widespread problem, and bodies' water requirements rise when fasting.

It is permissible to drink coffee or tea without sugar. You can even add a little cheese/ butter (bullet coffee as they call it in Keto diet). Dairy does not produce the same insulin response as carbs.

On OMAD days, I drink a few glasses of black coffee (expresso or Americano) at two/three-hour intervals. Coffee can help you lose weight by suppressing your appetite. Caffeine, a few hours before a meal, may release appetite hormones, and suppress feelings of hunger ([134]). Please consume coffee responsibly, as coffee contains caffeine, which can be very addicting if consumed in excess.

Believe me, hunger will not overcome you. You might feel hungry in the window when you usually eat (say, 9 a.m.), but after you cross that window with some water or caffeine, you won't feel hungry until the following window. Remember that we have conditioned our bodies to have many meals throughout the day, and our bodies are addicted to food.

What you may perceive as hunger is only a withdrawal symptom; once you have been accustomed to the fasting pattern, your body will automatically acclimate.

If you are still hungry, drink plenty of water, a little coffee (don't overdo the caffeine), green tea, masala tea (cinnamon, clove, cardamom, ginger), these elements decrease hunger and will definitely give you some time.

During the ketonic phase, we may lose bodily salts. To compensate for the salt loss, drink lemon juice with a pinch of salt.

As part of a healthy balanced diet, the first meal following fasting could be home prepared cuisine. There is no need to be concerned about nutrition or an extensive cuisine. Just be careful not to go overboard with UPF and sugar, since this can negate all the benefits you've gained from fasting.

Continue to follow your routine, if you are used to early morning walks/ runs or exercise, for example. There is no need to alter anything. In fact, you will reap significant benefits if you do mild activity during the fasting period, as it will aid in fat burning. If you want to conduct rigorous exercises during the fasting period (such as high intensity interval training or HIIT), consult your doctor or health practitioner.

It would be unfair to this chapter if I did not highlight certain disadvantages or side effects of fasting. Each person will react differently to fasting, but with time, the issues will fade and you will embrace it. Here are a few things to think about before fasting:

Hunger is the clearest symptom: your body and mind will need food at regular intervals. This will fade as you settle into your new eating regimen.

Digestive difficulties - During the fasting days, you may experience digestive issues. People also complain of constipation, especially after fasting for over 24 hours. Personally, this has only happened on the day after an OMAD and never during 16:8. This is not a significant problem; your bowel is simply acclimating to the change in the regimen and will settle down in no time. Constipation can also develop when not enough fiber is consumed during the feeding window.

Moodiness-Few people may have excessive moodiness, which includes a tendency to become irritated quickly. A drop in the blood sugar levels usually causes this. This is a recurrent problem that must be acknowledged and addressed. Irritability can be managed. The goal is to keep your mind active, away from food, and to believe in a greater purpose. We've all experienced it; sometimes we're so busy that we don't realise we've missed a few hours of eating; those who fast for religious reasons focus their minds on God (or a larger purpose) and are usually driven by a higher goal; these are some strategies to ease moodiness.

A little headache is a common fasting symptom. Low blood sugar levels, according to research, produce headaches while fasting for over 16 hours. In my experience, this is simply a withdrawal symptom. It goes away after a few days of fasting.

Improper fasting and feeding might cause malnutrition. If you fast carelessly and for an extended amount of time, or if you take fasting to extremes, you may suffer from malnutrition and other health concerns. Consuming UPF and sugar, for example, during the feeding window. It is critical that you maintain a balanced diet, which includes the foods you have been eating since childhood. We can restore calorie and nutrient requirements with a well-balanced diet. Get help if you are still in doubt. You can contact me if you require help (I have appended my contact details at the end of this book).

Clearly, fasting is an excellent way to lose weight and poses no substantial risks. However, if you have any underlying diseases such as diabetes, heart problems, senior citizens, children, being on medications, and so on, you should always visit your healthcare practitioner.

There is very little information on whether fasting poses any damage to women. Although fasting has no established negative effects on women, it is prudent to exercise caution and listen to your body. Fasting, unlike calorie-restricted diets, has no or very little disadvantage. If you don't like the idea or the methods, you may just return to your previous way of life, which is also totally safe. Fasting is an effective technique for weight loss and overall health. You should give it a shot.

If you have questions or require clarification on anything, feel free to reach out to me (I have appended my contact details at the end of this book).

I wish you the best of luck and success on your fasting adventure!

Chapter 8

Mind over body–"I" control YOU!

Chapter 8 - Mind over body: "I" control YOU!

When was the last time you had a strong craving to eat a cucumber or an orange? Yes, we all enjoy the flavor of an orange; however, have you ever craved one?

I don't want you, yet I can't abandon you! This has historically been my connection with sugar and energy-dense meals, including fries (let us call them energy-dense foods or EDF). Ice cream, pizza, fries, and cookies have been my go-to foods during my long evenings at the office. There have been days when I felt horrible and unforgiving of myself, often reeling with remorse. EDF has also been a fantastic stress reliever during times of emotional upheaval and unrelenting office space.

I've come dangerously near to having a nervous breakdown few times, and EDF rescued me emotionally many times. EDF has always been a source of conflict for me. I felt knowledge was the way out and did a nutrition certification course. I submerged myself in EDF resources and their detrimental effect.

Unfortunately, old habits die hard and knowledge can only take you so far; I was continually dragged into the EDF maelstrom and felt helpless. My body and mind refused to acknowledge the negative consequences.

Eventually, I learned that textbooks and certification could only carry me so far, and I found myself with more questions than when I began. Perhaps I am not an oddity, and many of you have had similar experiences.

Fortunately, you and I are not outliers; our proclivities are likely universal; we enjoy overindulgence, craving rich, calorie-dense foods while well aware that we "shouldn't" indulge. Worryingly, the awareness has little impact.

Our motivation to consume EDF extends beyond hunger and survival. I could go on and on about the benefits of germination, fermentation etc., but there is a propensity to gravitate toward foods that do us more harm than good. It's as though we craved EDF.

It's like trying to persuade a child to eat veggies and avoid chocolate. Yes, we can learn to eat nutritious food with information and some long-term training (habit building).

However, we all know that temptation to use EDF is constantly lurking around the corner; a colleague's birthday, a team lunch, a family/team get-together, a few difficult days at work, and wham, EDF engulfs you. You can only get so far with intellectual mastery and habit building. Your body and mind appear to collaborate to disobey and defeat you, much to your disappointment. Yes, we love fat, sugar, and carbohydrates, we shamelessly stuff ourselves at every opportunity.

Yes, there are a select few who have rigorously trained their mind and body over lengthy periods of time; they have failed many times and have somehow kept going. Our ancestral brain-gut circuitry is wired to gorge on high-calorie foods, which were once a scarce and treasured item.

Our brain's neurological circuits are tuned to reward us; dopamine, a feel-good hormone, is produced in the brain, triggering a cascade of responses that essentially makes you addicted to EDF.

We developed these mechanisms as a survival strategy where we feast during times of food abundance and fast during times of food scarcity. The issue is not with EDF, nor is it with us; rather, the issue may be with the environment in which we currently live.

Leave humans, even domestic animals, feast on treats, and any veterinarian would agree that pet obesity is a concern. According to research[135], obesity is even becoming a pandemic in pets. Owners have established an environment in which pets are continually rewarded. Owners feed the pets food meant for humans which is mostly UPF and sugar. They move less and are frequently confined to the four walls of the house. The only physical activity they have is short walks with their owners to answer nature's call.

Obesity affects not only pets, lab rats, hamsters, and pigs; there have also been reports of zoo animals becoming obese ([136]) Veterinarians advise pet owners to carefully monitor their pets' diets. Zoo animals' diets are meticulously balanced so that they do not gain weight. Yet, in the wild, the same animals are not obese.

Food abundance is so severe that even stray dogs in India are obese. The problem appears to be universal, and the problem is not with us, but with our surroundings or environment, which has been re-engineered and changed in such a way that it appears to be a one-way ticket to weight growth.

We are no different; we have developed to adapt to our surroundings through thousands and millions of years. when compared to our evolutionary history, the situation we find ourselves in now is new and only a fraction of a second old. We are not in our natural habitat. The artificial environments we've built are convenient for us. For no apparent reason, we continue to reward and indulge in ourselves. We are quietly digging a hole for ourselves. We already know that the EDF appeals to our brain's reward centre, and corporations are well aware of this. When our brain is rewarded by these meals, the habit is reinforced, and our brain coaxes us to continue pursuing the reward.

Our brain intricately relates a specific scenario to a specific food (coke during a football game, eating out on weekends, Pizza and cola during team party/ after programme launch or late-night working/ stressful events, desert after lunch, evening snacking at the café with colleagues, and so on), and habit is reinforced with repetition.

Everyone nowadays is on a calorie-restricted diet. We wish to lose weight through calorie restricting or by eliminating particular EDFs, such as chocolate or ice cream. As previously said, EDF addiction is a conditioned habit in which we have repeatedly educated our mind and body to ingest EDF under specific conditions. Is it possible to eliminate cravings through mindful calorie restriction? The answer - yes and no!

Short-term calorie restriction has been demonstrated in studies to increase desire. Long-term restrained eaters' profit because they can resist temptation for longer. Long-term dieters can condition themselves away from cravings. However, a long-term diet is arduous and difficult to sustain. Weight-loss studies in obese people consistently show that calorie restriction reduces food cravings. This could be because of the process of elimination, in which we can detach craving from an event and replace it with healthier options. Let me emphasise this point once more. According to another study,[137] habit is one of the most powerful predictors of eating behavior.

- We don't need a lot of information to

determine when something is a habit, according to this study.

- Simply intending to break the habit is a poor predictor of success.
- Situational factors, not only hunger, activate our eating behaviors.

So, rather than dieting, the key is to unlearn the habit or decouple the urge. With this in mind, let us look for ways and means to avoid sugar (or EDF).

Proximity—In most circumstances, we end up nibbling at home. We are used to stacking our refrigerator and shelves with EDF. To unlearn this pattern, we should practice mindful purchasing and make a conscious decision to avoid purchasing EDF from the grocery shop. If you buy bakery items or prefer a specific bakery or brand, I propose taking an alternative route and avoiding the temptation to buy altogether. A bakery is only one example. Extend this to any EDF temptation, such as avoiding McDonald's or a supermarket aisle, for example.

This may appear tough at first, but with practice, you should be able to train your mind, and the brain will quickly move into autopilot mode. Developing the practice of avoiding unconscious traps and purchasing junk food places no burden on your willpower when compared with buying and then controlling the temptation to eat.

The less junk you have at your home, the less is the tendency to consume. Our mind longs for instant gratification and will grab something within reach rather than moving out finding an EDF in the grocery store or ordering online. Within no time, the habit of purchasing junk foods will gradually fade, as will the practice of junking. We may occasionally wind up snacking in the office cafeteria. Avoiding the cafeteria is the simplest approach. However, this is easier said than done. We must adapt to society, and you may feel forced to say no to a friend. If you can't avoid it, select a healthy choice (such a salad or fruits); in the short run, the temptation will be overwhelming. However, temptation will fade with time as you have trained your mind to choose healthy alternatives.

Similarity- we want certain meals in specific settings (such as popcorn while watching a movie in a theater). One option is to exert control over it, if not totally avoid. In such circumstances, instead of nibbling during this time, opt for a healthy choice. When we are in a scenario, we usually make split-second decisions. Another option is to pause, wait a few minutes, and think about it before purchasing the snack. It is difficult to decouple similarity bias though. However, if you can devote a reasonable period, it will work.

Find a buddy-If everything fails, you might find a buddy who has a similar goal to you and who supports or works alongside you so that you can motivate each other. The company we keep sometimes influences our eating habits and intake habits we keep. What would happen, for example, if you were dining with a glutenous or overindulgent friend? We may wind up pampering ourselves, whether deliberately or unknowingly. Alternatively, at your friend's request, we may wind up having the extra dessert. Consider sharing a meal with an underweight friend who hasn't established an appetite, would you binge/overindulge in his presence?

According to studies,[138] people look outward for signs of their surroundings to choose when to stop eating. Obesity may increase because of our intrinsic urge to imprint others or an attempt to comply. We hang around with obese people and end up indulging inadvertently. To be sure, our eating habits are influenced in the long run by our familiarity with the companion and the same goals we share. You should pick an eating companion who sets a good example, shares a common aim, and is reasonable.

4. The Stranger paradox —Finding a buddy was difficult for me. All said and done, we are a people with distinct personalities and upbringing. Twinning with someone would always present a distinct problem. I then met a mentor, who was a complete stranger. Our interactions were rational and nonjudgmental. My mentor educated me about diet, calories, and so on, but he eventually relinquished control over me. "Who am

I?" He used to ask. "I'm just a beacon of light. You are the ship's commander." We eventually agreed that I could eat whatever I wanted, and he never interfered. He never claimed this food was correct, or that was incorrect. He would only respond if asked. To be honest, there came a point when I realised what I needed to do to reach the goal. My mentor served as an anchor. We agreed I would photograph the food I eat every day, every meal and drink and share it with him. He promised me he would be completely impartial and would only look at the photo and provide a recommendation if I asked for it. That my mentor would actually see what I ate at each meal was the deciding factor. All I had to do was get the bravery to tell what I ate at each meal. Yes, there was some hesitation at first. However, fact that you are sharing the image for a greater good kept me going. Something spectacular happened when I started sharing the photos. I instinctively wanted to share a picture of an EDF free plate, every time I felt the urge to snack, the fact that I should share with him actually stopped me. Slowly but steadily, my plate became healthier, more balanced, and my snacking was substantially reduced. Just because someone is watching what you eat was enough to cause a difference. It's like wearing a shabby dress and walking into a room full of strangers. We realise the person opposite is a complete stranger, and we do not know what he is thinking, and honestly, it doesn't matter what I wear; and yet we want to appear presentable, so we dress appropriately for an occasion.

Similarly, even though I knew my mentor didn't judge, I still wanted my dish to look decent. Every time I ate, I ate the healthier option rather than the EDF. It took some time, but I've finally broken free from my bad habits. I am not dependent on EDF. I do occasionally cheat, but I am not hooked. I'm still not sure why sharing the photos with a complete stranger worked so well. Instead, I could have shared it with my friends and family. According to one study, eating with friends increases an individual's[139] energy consumption by up to 18% when compared to eating with strangers.

And this sealed the deal. I could get into a mental place where I was confident that the individual would not judge me, make jokes about me, or make fun of me in front of common friends. I strongly advise you to share images with a mentor or a complete stranger.

It works, believe me. If you cannot locate a stranger/mentor, please contact me and I can make suitable arrangements (I have appended my contact details at the end of this book, please feel free to reach out, subscribe to the program and derive immense benefits).

Stress reliever:

The Mind and body are inextricably linked, with each influencing the other. When you become furious, your heart rate increases, your blood pressure rises, your eyes dilate, your muscles twitch, your facial expression changes, your posture becomes aggressive, and your breathing pattern alters. Your body prepares for a conflict, and your concentration narrows and focuses on the individual or the situation to the exclusion of all else.

Almost all of us have experienced these changes; we may not have been aware of them, but the physiological changes caused by emotion are indisputable. And the converse is also true: a simple chuckle or even artificially smiling or holding your partner's hand relieves our aggression, cuddling, a few deep breaths calms our racing heart, slows our breathing, relaxes our body and mind, and we wonder why we became furious.

Our autonomic nerve system, or ANS, is the source of this relationship. This is your surveillance system, which constantly monitors for impending danger and guides you to safety. When we receive danger cues, it allows us to react swiftly, such as seeing a snake on the walk, and it also allows us to relax, such as a child in his or her parents' arms.

The sympathetic nervous system and the parasympathetic nervous system make up the autonomic nervous system.

The sympathetic nervous system (SNS) regulates our flight-fight-freeze responses in response to a specific event, such as encountering a snake (freeze, faint or shutdown) or a predator (flight) or during an altercation (fight).

The parasympathetic nervous system (PNS) acts as a counterbalance, relaxing and reassuring us. Typically, these two systems cooperate and balance each other out. The ability to balance the two is critical to your general health and well-being.

Aside from the PNS and SNS, the ANS encompasses another component called the enteric nervous system, which is important in digestion and is also known as the gut brain nexus. Nature created the ANS as a survival system to protect us from injury and danger over millions of years of evolution.

The ANS exerts impact on the body at multiple levels, including digestion, circulatory, immunological, muscles, and skeleton, among others, with the primary goal of preparing you for impending danger or shutting down in the event of an impending unmanageable hazard.

It is named the autonomic (involuntary or unconscious) system for a reason: respiration, heartbeat, digestion, and so on are not under our active control. Controlling our respiration, heart rate, and digestion at all times would have been a monumental feat.

When the ANS is on high alert, your body and mind

work together to combat the threat. We are hard-wired to search for hazards, threats can be real or imaginary. The ANS is essentially a safety net for you, with the ultimate purpose of your survival against all odds. The ANS exerts control over you via a nerve known as the vagus nerve (or the wandering nerve), this nerve runs from the tip of your brain to your abdomen, passing through many vital organs along the route.

During times of stress or worry, the vagus nerve causes your heart to race, your breathing to shallow, and you to feel butterflies in your stomach. The vagus nerve controls your internal organs. While the intricate brain and physiological circulatory system works perfectly well for actual threats, things get complicated when the mind perceives a threat (phantom threat), and the balance is pushed to where we end up in free fall.

Stress is one of the most serious perceived risks to the modern human. It is not about minor concerns, such as interview nerves or working on deadlines; rather, I am referring to the all-encompassing worry that consumes our mind and body daily. As we are conditioned for stress, tension becomes innate and emerges in various forms and surfaces for no reason.

We've all heard and read about the negative effects of stress, and the list is long. We also know that weight increase is one of them. However, we downplay the effect of stress on weight gain.

The common misconception about stress and weight gain is that we binge when we are stressed, that calorie dense food relieves stress, that we eat more when we are stressed, and that therefore we gain weight. Yes, stress increases the want to eat EDF; ironically, when we are under chronic stress, we gain weight even if we do not binge or consume calorie-dense foods. Are you Wondering how? Let's find out.

Stress activates a series of chemical and hormonal pathways that include adrenaline, CRH, and cortisol. These hormones are necessary for your brain and body to deal with the perceived threat. Adrenaline actually makes you feel less hungry by shifting your attention away from digestion and toward your muscles, where the goal is to prepare you for flight. The Cortisol is still in the body after the threat has passed.

Cortisol is a glucocorticoid hormone that is generated from cholesterol. The adrenal glands, which are on top of the kidneys produce cortisol.

Cortisol is released for a variety of causes, including waking up promptly in the morning (described in the fasting chapter), physical exertion, and so on.

Cortisol normally functions as follows in times of [140]stress:

1. The mind detects a threat.

2. The sympathetic nervous system is stimulated, and a

complex cocktail of chemicals, including adrenaline and cortisol, is released.

3. The body is preparing for a fight-flight-freeze. The body now requires a burst of energy to leave the threat, therefore a burst of glucose is released.

4. We know that insulin stops fat burning and initiates fat storage. Cortisol however does not want the body to store glucose as fat because it requires an immediate surge of energy. Cortisol suppresses insulin synthesis.

5.As the heart rate rises, breathing shallows, and blood rushes through the veins, the body is now ready for flight or fight.

6.The threat has passed, and hormone levels automatically return to normal.

While this works perfectly for actual threats, things go out of balance in situation of chronic stress as persistent stress results in cortisol overload. Long-term cortisol exposure can wreak havoc on your system, causing sadness, anxiety, cardiac problems, and obesity. The question is, how can cortisol cause us to gain weight?

Insulin resistance-While research on this topic is still ongoing, a few studies ([141], [142]) have showed that high cortisol levels lead to insulin resistance. Sustained cortisol levels would cause sugar increases and insulin inhibition. Over time, the cells that consume glucose wear out, requiring the pancreas to release more insulin to drive glucose into the cells. As blood glucose levels remain high, the pancreas goes into overdrive and tries to keep up with insulin demand. Overtime, insulin resistance develops in cells. As cortisol levels remain high, this creates a vicious cycle. In the insulin chapter, we previously discussed the dangers of insulin resistance.

Gaining weight and distributing fat- According to this [143]study, cortisol has a direct influence on fat accumulation and weight increase in stressed persons because of the production of certain enzymes that lead to obesity. Sustained cortisol levels affect fat distribution, causing fat to be stored in a deep abdomen, which, if unchecked, can lead to obesity[144].

Cortisol causes overeating- Consistently high glucose levels and insulin blockage cause cells to be starved of glucose in areas where they need energy. As one technique for providing energy to previously starving cells, the body sends hunger signals to the brain. As a result, we have more appetite[145] and, it gets difficult to resist craving since glucose-depleted cells drive us to binge on EDF. Cortisol also interferes with the hormone[146] that regulates satiety, resulting in typical stress bingeing behavior.

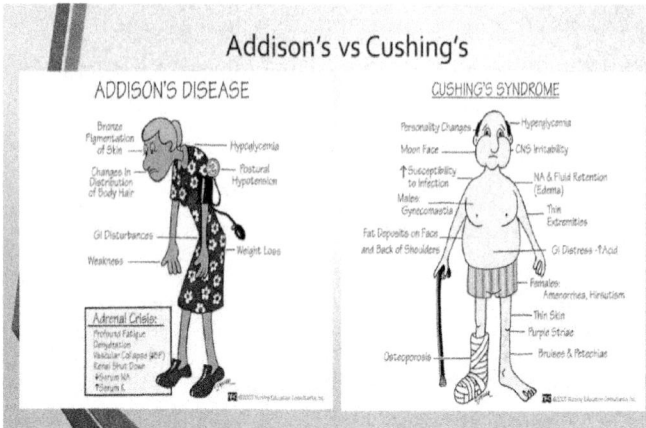

Addison's vs Cushing's

ADDISON'S DISEASE

Bronze
Pigmentation
of Skin

Changes In
Distribution
of Body Hair

GI Disturbances

Weakness

Hypoglycemia

Postural
Hypotension

Weight Loss

Adrenal Crisis:
Profound Fatigue
Dehydration
Vascular Collapse (↓BP)
Renal Shut Down
↓Serum Na
↑Serum K

CUSHING'S SYNDROME

Personality Changes

Moon Face

↑Susceptibility
to Infection
Males:
Gynecomastia

Fat Deposits on Face
and Back of Shoulders

Osteoporosis

Hyperglycemia

CNS Irritability

NA & Fluid Retention
(Edema)

Thin
Extremities

GI Distress - ↑Acid

Females:
Amenorrhea, Hirsutism

Thin Skin

Purple Striae

Bruises & Petechiae

Image - Quizlet

Two classic examples of how cortisol directly impacts weight gain is Cushing's syndrome and Addisons Disease. Cushing's syndrome, a condition caused by having too much cortisol in your body resulting in persistently raised glucose levels, which result in weight gain, high blood sugar, and insulin resistance. Addisons Disease occurs when the body does not create enough cortisol[147]. Rapid/significant weight loss, loss of appetite, and low blood sugar levels are all hallmark symptoms of Addison's disease.

As a result, the iconic calorie restriction diets have been defeated. Instead of addressing the major problem, which is stress, we continue to focus on trendy diets. Satiety and appetite are out of control because of high cortisol levels. It becomes impossible to control calories, and you end up bingeing, creating even more stress and anguish. Short-term dieting will lose out in the long run.

We don't get thinner or healthier by limiting carbs, fats, or exercising, since the body will eventually triumph; will power is frequently exaggerated. Cortisol, like insulin, is a blessing and a curse. Sustained high cortisol levels cause rapid weight gain and a shift in fat distribution.

So, what is the solution? Let us return to ANS. The key to stress reduction is ANS modulation. We may ease it if we discover how your body reacts to dangers. As we all know, the sympathetic nervous system causes stress, whereas the parasympathetic nervous system immediately steps in and calms the body during times of normalcy. The sympathetic nervous system has the upper hand while under stress. We need to activate the parasympathetic nervous system.

One of the key branches of the parasympathetic nervous system is the vagus Nerve. The vagus nerve is the one that disrupts the sympathetic nervous system and causes stress.

The main reason we feel safer and more normal is because of the vagus nerve. Vagus nerve reduces tension, promotes relaxation, and create a sense of security. How do we stimulate the vagus nerve, then?

Breathing-The simple process of deep breathing and

slowly exhaling generates a response from the vagus Nerve. Deep breathing activates the relaxation pathways and quickly restores semblance. We always understood this, but it's difficult to recall and adjust in times of crisis.

The Sympathetic nervous system elicits shallow breathing, whereas focused deep breathing should stimulate the Parasympathetic nervous system. There are many breathing techniques; however, select an excellent teacher to get the most appropriate approach.

Meditation:

Practice awareness and meditation. Again, there are many materials on mindfulness and meditation. Mindfulness should not be limited to a specific time of day; you can instill mindfulness at various levels such as slow purposeful eating, walking, engaging walks, sitting in a café with a loved one and having a drink, reading a book, gardening, painting, drawing, dancing, doing yoga, playing a sport you enjoy, cooking, and so on.

Awareness and positive thinking with a purpose- Our brain is continually on the lookout for potential hazards. When it detects a threat, it will gravitate toward it, resulting in an endless cycle of negative self-talk. If our mind can think negatively, it can think positively. When we develop a positive attitude and make it a habit not to feel scared by threats by engaging in continual positive thinking. Stress and anxiety fade away quickly.

Smoking and weight[148]:

To keep a slender figure
No one can deny...

Reach for a LUCKY instead of a sweet

LUCKY STRIKE "IT'S TOASTED" CIGARETTES

"It's toasted"
No Throat Irritation-No Cough.

Smokers share a strange relationship with weight. Cigarrete was considered a potent weight loss therapy and was heavily advertised during the 19th century. Even today, some people who are trying to reduce their body fat believe that they have found the weight-loss medication (just google and you will find resources). It does not require a prescription, it is inexpensive, are within reasonable ranges for most people.

The chemical in question is nicotine, and when it is introduced into the body, it suppresses craving for energy dense food, increases energy expenditure, lessens the frequency with which one snacks, and causes weight loss. The increase in energy expenditure is significant as it can cause the loss of 10 kg in body weight over 1 year. Nicotine effects regulation of both eating and energy expenditure.

Researchers have known for a long time that smokers' weigh less than nonsmokers, and most smokers who stop smoking, gain weight when they do.

Data show that smoking slows the weight gain that comes with getting older. This makes the difference in weight between smokers and nonsmokers who gain weight over time, but it goes away when smokers quit. Weight gain is an obvious side effect for people who quit smoking. On average, smokers weigh 4–5 kg less than people who don't smoke. People who stop smoking gain, on average, 4.5 kg in the 6–12 months after they stop. Some smokers who are predisposed for weight gain end up gaining much more weight after quitting (as much as 10 kg).

When people stop smoking, they lose the boost to their metabolism and the way nicotine makes them feel full.

This can cause them to eat more calories and this makes people gain weight.

Many people, especially women, have used smoking to control their appetite, and they say that the fear of gaining a lot of weight when they quit is one of the main reasons they keep smoking despite the health risks. There is a new trend of using electronic cigarettes (i.e., vaping) to lose weight. The internet is full of stories about how vaping makes people feel less hungry. Vaping is considered a safer alternative to smoking as it is potentially less cancer causing. Now, before you think that smoking or vaping could be a drug that helps you lose weight, keep reading.

1. Cigarette smoke is very poisonous, which is why half of people who smoke for their whole lives die young.
2. Smokers have more visceral fat compared with total fat, so their waist-to-hip ratio is higher than that of nonsmokers.
3. Changes in body composition, like more visceral fat, are linked to insulin resistance.
4. Nicotine is not a safe substance, no matter how it gets into the body (cigarettes or vaping), and it has a very high chance of making someone addicted.
5. Smoking/ vaping is not a magic pill, that will help you lose weight. The weight loss comes with a cost: you have to keep vaping forever to

keep the weight off, and you also get hooked on nicotine.

Bottomline - Stop smoking, the risk of smoking by far outweighs the benefits.

Chapter 9

Tenets–Take one step at a time!

Chapter 9 – Tenets: Take one step at a time!

Remember that your mind is a formidable foe, your brain and body behave as if they don't care about you. That's why they don't care about your weight-loss aim, which may give you the impression that they're working against you. Even while you may believe that you have total control over your thoughts, you actually have very little control over the decisions you unconsciously make when you are around food.

The human body puts on weight and keeps it there under all circumstances. Our very existence depends on it. As long as we reject this scientific fact, we can never achieve and maintain a healthy weight.

You should be very careful, take tiny steps and train your mind and body slowly.

Begin with simple, healthful behaviors that you can gradually expand on. The only way to lose weight and keep it off is to make a permanent switch to healthier foods. This will transmit signals to your brain, assisting you in losing weight healthily. Pay focus on the task at hand rather than the number. If you find that a new habit isn't working for you, switch to something simpler. The goal should not be to maintain a specific weight, but to remain healthy and fit.

Admittedly, we intuitively knew that we should eat healthy, stay away from sugar and processed food, don't get stressed etc., you are now equipped with the knowledge of how the mind and the body works, the affect various food has on us.

let's culminate this book with clear rules you should follow to manage weight and lead a fulfilling and healthy life.

Rule 1: Eat healthy

- The easiest lifestyle change is to consume what your grandmother used to consume. Our forefathers' diet was balanced for your body type and the environment. It does not matter whether your forefathers were vegetarians or non-vegetarians.
- Consume home cooked food at all times.
- All carbohydrates are not made same, fill your plate with whole real unprocessed foods, whole grains, green leafy vegetables, fruits, whole grains, beans, nuts, seeds, olive oil, organic, range, or grass-fed animal products (poultry, lamb, beef, pork, eggs), and wild, smaller fish such as salmon.
- Consume seasonally and locally available food.
- Your plate should be colorful. The key is to eat a variety of foods, and the microbes in your gut love variety. A healthy gut microbiota will

definitely help you stay at a healthy weight.

- The unassuming superfood is resistant starch, and you should eat more pulses and raw fruits.
- Rice and wheat should be safe to eat in moderation, unless you have a health problem or your doctor tells you otherwise.
- Consume ample natural protein (plant or animal based).
- Consume fat in moderation. Do not worry about saturated, unsaturated fats.
- Read labels carefully.
- Consume dairy in moderation unless you have a health problem or your doctor tells you otherwise.
- Inculcate fermentation techniques of your ancestors. Fermented foods have significant health benefits.
- Have sprouts, it is a superfood.
- Consume locally available millets, they are a significant source of fiber and resistant starch.
- Inculcate habit of consuming apple cider vinegar.
- Consume free range meat and organ meat if you are an omnivore.
- Inculcate the habit of mindful purchasing and consuming.
- Practice deep breathing and meditation.
- Body is built to move, get up and move.

Practice micro exercises.

- Find a buddy, a mentor.

Rule 2: Control Unhealthy

- Learn to identify trigger foods. For some of us, just one slice of pizza has the power to send us into a downward spiral of overeating. Not just processed, sugary meals and beverages can act as triggers.
- Drastically reduce consumption of white sugar and white flour.
- Consume white rice in moderation.
- Reduce ultra-processed food.
- Do not consume processed meat.
- Do not have multiple meals a day.
- Fruit juice is not healthy.
- Be careful with fructose.
- Quit smoking, beware of post smoking weight gain.
- Don't overdo protein.
- Trans fat–Be careful.
- Limit consuming outside food only for special occasions.

Rule 3: Increase fasting window

- Fasting is supreme medicine, it is safe to skip meals (especially breakfast). Consult your doctor if you have any underlying health issues.

Rule 4: Manage stress

- Manage stress, meditate, practice breathing techniques, sleep well. Seek support if things get overwhelming.

Rule 5: Move

- Body is built to move, get up and move.
- Practice micro exercises.

Rule 6: Never diet

- Ironically, why many diets work initially is because it recommends tenet 1 and 2.
- Don't count calories, don't do calorie restriction diet.

Rule 7: Listen to your body

- Never follow a rule blindly, always listen to your body.
- If you are thirsty, drink water. If you are hungry, eat whole foods.
- Remember cravings and biases. Try your best not to get sucked into biases.

Rule 8: Repeat Rules 1 to 7!

The first step in any journey is to understand and accept that mistakes will be made. It will be hard. We might not commit to it the way we want, and we might not get the results we were hoping for. If we keep putting things off and never even take the first step, the new year's or birthday resolutions we made never come true.

Don't be hard on yourself when things get hard. Like you would be a close friend or family member, be kind and patient with yourself. How would you act if one of your brothers or sisters told you they were having a hard time? would you scold them, call them names, make them feel worse about themselves, or make them frown even more?

One of the hardest parts of your journey is to stick to the methods, focus on the process and not the results, keep going even when it seems impossible, and be kind to yourself when you slip up and don't follow the process. We all make mistakes, and sometimes we repeat the same ones on purpose. This makes us human; our flaws show we aren't perfect, so let's stop trying to be perfect. What does your inner voice tell you when you can't stick to a diet, binge, etc.? We are getting farther away from ourselves by teaching and encouraging thoughts that hurt us, our self-esteem takes a hit when we talk to ourselves in a way that makes us feel bad about ourselves. We stop looking inside and start seeking support outside. When you're depressed, your mind likes to binge and lose control. It makes you want to run away from reality, and before you know it, you're in a downward spiral. All the hard work you've done for months may seem like nothing.

You can't get out of the inner whirlpool because it takes up your whole body.

You need to get back in touch with your true self and take back what is yours and what you deserve. Try to be kind to yourself.

I sometimes think that instead of calling it our inner voice, we should treat it more like our inner child. What would you say to a scared or worried child? In the same way, what would you tell your inner child who thinks she can't commit to something because she failed at it before or more than once? You would tell your inner voice, "It's okay that you missed it this time. There's always next time. Try to be careful next time, maybe take a moment to think before deciding, etc." you would talk to your inner voice like a child. Children make mistakes, and sometimes they do them on purpose. instead of calling them names and punishing them, you show them love. Think of them as a soft feather brushing against a fine glass.

Tell yourself that the way you are is fine. there is always room to get better. I'm different from everyone else, so why should I compare myself to them? Yes, I made a mistake this time, but next time I'll be more careful. This doesn't mean that you won't keep getting worse and worse. it will, however, keep you from falling into a deep hole repeatedly. And it won't take long or many tries before you can find the abyss and stay away from it. You figure out how to deal with your inner child.

Remember that the only person you should be kind to is yourself. Make peace with yourself, and you'll be on your way to reaching your goals. Don't find a quick fix; instead, take small steps. We can't lose the weight we've gained over months and years in just a few days or weeks. Give it some time and don't hurt yourself.

If you think you can't get out on your own, ask for help. Practice mindfulness and take one of the many self-compassion courses that are easy to find. Again, there are free apps, YouTube videos, and a lot of other online resources. Everything is there. You just need to look at the right spot. Reach out to me in case you need any support. I wish you all the best in your journey.

Thank you.

<Notes>

<Notes>

<Notes>

<Notes>

<Notes>

<Notes>

1 Contact details

Arun Rao

Email - guilt.free@outlook.com

Phone (WhatsApp messages only) - +44 7776815301 or +44 7776815294

WhatsApp group invite –

Click on this link -

https://chat.whatsapp.com/C2gGuNfbncHBLaf6im0lnC

Scan QR Code to join the group –

2 Contact and subscription link

Email - Guilt.free@outlook.com

Phone (WhatsApp messages only) - +44 7776815301

WhatsApp group invite –

Click on this link -

https://chat.whatsapp.com/C2gGuNfbncHBLaf6im0lnC

Scan QR Code –

[3]Klok, M., Jakobsdottir, S., & Drent, M. (2006). The role of leptin and ghrelin in the regulation of food intake and body weight in humans: A review. Obesity Reviews, 8, 21-34.

[4] Müller, M., Bosy-Westphal, A., & Heymsfield, S. (2010). F1000Reports,

[5] The Effects of Exercise and Physical Activity on Weight Loss

and Maintenance." The Effects of Exercise and Physical Activity on Weight Loss and Maintenance - ScienceDirect, 9 July 2018, ww.sciencedirect.com/science/article/abs/pii/S0033062018301 440.

[6] "Weight-Loss Outcomes: A Systematic Review and Meta-Analysis of Weight-Loss Clinical Trials with a Minimum 1-Year Follow-up - PubMed." PubMed, 1 Oct. 2007, pubmed.ncbi.nlm.nih.gov/17904936.

[7] Donnelly, Joseph E., et al. "Aerobic Exercise Alone Results in Clinically Significant Weight Loss for Men and Women: Midwest Exercise Trial-2 - PMC." PubMed Central (PMC), www.ncbi.nlm.nih.gov/pmc/articles/PMC3630467. Accessed 11 Sept. 2022

[8] Appetite Control and Energy Balance: Impact of Exercise - PubMed." PubMed, 1 Feb. 2015, pubmed.ncbi.nlm.nih.gov/25614205

[9] Consumption of Ultra-Processed Foods and Obesity in Canada - PubMed." PubMed, 1 Feb. 2019, pubmed.ncbi.nlm.nih.gov/30238324/

[10] Poti, Jennifer M., et al. "Ultra-Processed Food Intake and Obesity: What Really Matters for Health – Processing or Nutrient Content? - PMC." PubMed Central (PMC), www.ncbi.nlm.nih.gov/pmc/articles/PMC5787353. Accessed 11 Sept. 2022

[11] Resolved: There Is Sufficient Scientific Evidence That Decreasing Sugar-Sweetened Beverage Consumption Will Reduce

the Prevalence of Obesity and Obesity-Related Diseases - PubMed." PubMed, 1 Aug. 2013, pubmed.ncbi.nlm.nih.gov/23763695.

[12] Stern, Dalia, et al. "Changes in Sugar-Sweetened Soda Consumption, Weight, and Waist Circumference: 2-Year Cohort of Mexican Women - PMC." PubMed Central (PMC), 1 Nov. 2017, www.ncbi.nlm.nih.gov/pmc/articles/PMC5637666.

[13] "How Dieting Makes the Lean Fatter: From a Perspective of Body Composition Autoregulation through Adipostats and Proteinstats Awaiting Discovery - PubMed." PubMed, 1 Feb. 2015, pubmed.ncbi.nlm.nih.gov/25614201. /

[14] "Energy Balance and Obesity: What Are the Main Drivers? - PubMed." PubMed, 1 Mar. 2017, pubmed.ncbi.nlm.nih.gov/28210884. /

[15] https://pubmed.ncbi.nlm.nih.gov/24986822/

[16] Eliasson, Björn, et al. "Cephalic Phase of Insulin Secretion in Response to a Meal Is Unrelated to Family History of Type 2 Diabetes - PMC." PubMed Central (PMC), 13 Mar. 2017, www.ncbi.nlm.nih.gov/pmc/articles/PMC5348013 /

[17] Obesity and Overweight." Obesity and Overweight, 9 June 2021, www.who.int/news-room/fact-sheets/detail/obesity-and-overweight.

[18] Obesity and Overweight." Obesity and Overweight, 9 June 2021, www.who.int/news-room/fact-sheets/detail/obesity-and-overweight.

[19] "About Sugar | International Sugar Organization." About Sugar | International Sugar Organization, www.isosugar.org/sugarsector/sugar.

[20] DiNicolantonio, James J., and James H. OKeefe. "Added Sugars Drive Coronary Heart Disease via Insulin Resistance and Hyperinsulinaemia: A New Paradigm - PMC." PubMed Central (PMC), 29 Nov. 2017, www.ncbi.nlm.nih.gov/pmc/articles/PMC5708308.

[21] Chronic Hyperglycemia and Glucose Toxicity: Pathology and Clinical Sequelae - PubMed." PubMed, 1 Nov. 2012, pubmed.ncbi.nlm.nih.gov/23322142/

[22] Luger, Maria, et al. "Sugar-Sweetened Beverages and Weight Gain in Children and Adults: A Systematic Review from 2013 to 2015 and a Comparison with Previous Studies - PMC." PubMed Central (PMC), 14 Dec. 2017, www.ncbi.nlm.nih.gov/pmc/articles/PMC5836186.

[23] Vos, Miriam B., et al. "Added Sugars and Cardiovascular Disease Risk in Children: A Scientific Statement From the American Heart Association." PubMed Central (PMC), 22 Aug. 2016, www.ncbi.nlm.nih.gov/pmc/articles/PMC5365373

[24] https://onlinelibrary.wiley.com/doi/full/10.1111/j.1360-0443.2011.03373.x?referringRepId=25149

[25] Vos, Miriam B., et al. "Added Sugars and Cardiovascular Disease Risk in Children: A Scientific Statement From the American Heart Association." PubMed Central (PMC), 22 Aug.

2016, www.ncbi.nlm.nih.gov/pmc/articles/PMC5365373

[26] Vos, Miriam B., et al. "Added Sugars and Cardiovascular Disease Risk in Children: A Scientific Statement From the American Heart Association." PubMed Central (PMC), 22 Aug. 2016, www.ncbi.nlm.nih.gov/pmc/articles/PMC5365373

[27] "Scientific Opinion on the Substantiation of Health Claims Related to Fructose and Reduction of Post-Prandial Glycaemic Responses (ID 558) Pursuant to Article 213(1) of Regulation (EC) No 1924/2006 | EFSA." European Food Safety Authority, 30 June 2011, www.efsa.europa.eu/en/efsajournal/pub/2223

[28] Parks, Elizabeth J., et al. "Dietary Sugars Stimulate Fatty Acid Synthesis in Adults." PubMed Central (PMC), www.ncbi.nlm.nih.gov/pmc/articles/PMC2546703. Accessed 11 Sept. 2022.

[29] https://data.worldobesity.org/tables/ranking-obesity-by-country-adults-1.pdf?

[30] Qin, Junjie, et al. "A Human Gut Microbial Gene Catalog Established by Metagenomic Sequencing - PMC." PubMed Central (PMC), www.ncbi.nlm.nih.gov/pmc/articles/PMC3779803

[31] Martinez, Jason E., et al. "Frontiers | Unhealthy Lifestyle and Gut Dysbiosis: A Better Understanding of the Effects of Poor Diet and Nicotine on the Intestinal Microbiome." Frontiers, 1 Jan. 2001, www.frontiersin.org/articles/10.3389/fendo.2021.667066/full.

[32] Martinez, Jason E., et al. "Frontiers | Unhealthy Lifestyle and

Gut Dysbiosis: A Better Understanding of the Effects of Poor Diet and Nicotine on the Intestinal Microbiome." Frontiers, 1 Jan. 2001,

www.frontiersin.org/articles/10.3389/fendo.2021.667066/full.

[33] "Antibiotics in Early Life and Obesity - PubMed." PubMed, 1 Mar. 2015, pubmed.ncbi.nlm.nih.gov/25488483.

[34] Davis, Cindy D. "The Gut Microbiome and Its Role in Obesity - PMC." PubMed Central (PMC), www.ncbi.nlm.nih.gov/pmc/articles/PMC5082693. Accessed 11 Sept. 2022.

[35] Davis, Cindy D. "The Gut Microbiome and Its Role in Obesity - PMC." PubMed Central (PMC), www.ncbi.nlm.nih.gov/pmc/articles/PMC5082693. Accessed 11 Sept. 2022.

[36] Classification and Measurement of Nutritionally Important Starch Fractions - PubMed." PubMed, 1 Oct. 1992, pubmed.ncbi.nlm.nih.gov/1330528/

[37] Silva, Ygor Parladore, et al. "Frontiers | The Role of Short-Chain Fatty Acids From Gut Microbiota in Gut-Brain Communication." Frontiers, 1 Jan. 2001, www.frontiersin.org/articles/10.3389/fendo.2020.00025/full

[38] Silva, Ygor Parladore, et al. "Frontiers | The Role of Short-Chain Fatty Acids From Gut Microbiota in Gut-Brain Communication." Frontiers, 1 Jan. 2001, www.frontiersin.org/articles/10.3389/fendo.2020.00025/full

39 "Insulin-Sensitizing Effects of Dietary Resistant Starch and

Effects on Skeletal Muscle and Adipose Tissue Metabolism - PubMed." PubMed, 1 Sept. 2005, pubmed.ncbi.nlm.nih.gov/16155268/ and "Resistant Starch from High-Amylose Maize Increases Insulin Sensitivity in Overweight and Obese Men - PubMed." PubMed, 1 Apr. 2012, pubmed.ncbi.nlm.nih.gov/22357745

[40] "Insulin-Sensitizing Effects of Dietary Resistant Starch and Effects on Skeletal Muscle and Adipose Tissue Metabolism - PubMed." PubMed, 1 Sept. 2005, pubmed.ncbi.nlm.nih.gov/16155268. and "Resistant Starch from High-Amylose Maize Increases Insulin Sensitivity in Overweight and Obese Men - PubMed." PubMed, 1 Apr. 2012, pubmed.ncbi.nlm.nih.gov/22357745

[41]

https://www.sciencedirect.com/science/article/abs/pii/S01448 61799001472

[42] Eroglu EI, Buyuktuncer Z. The effect of various cooking methods on resistant starch content of foods. Nutrition and Food Science. 2017;47(4):522-533. DOI: 10.1371/journal.pone.0182604

[43] Eroglu EI, Buyuktuncer Z. The effect of various cooking methods on resistant starch content of foods. Nutrition and Food Science. 2017;47(4):522-533. DOI: 10.1371/journal.pone.0182604

[44] Juárez-García E, Agama-Acevedo E, SăyagoAyerdi SG, Rodrǐguez-Ambriz SL, Bello-Pěrez LA. Composition, digestibility

and application in breadmaking of banana flour. Plant Foods for Human Nutrition. 2006;61:131-137. DOI: 10.1007/s11130-006-0020-x

[46] Ho L-H, Noor Aziah AA, Bhat R. Mineral composition and pasting properties of banana pseudo-stem flour from Musa acuminata x balbisiana cv. Awak grown locally in Perak, Malaysia. International Food Research Journal. 2012;19(2):409-416

47 Sajilata MG, Siigbal RS, Kulkarmi PR. Resistant starch—A review. Food Science and Food Safety. 2006;5:1-17. DOI: 10.1111/j.1541-4337.2006.tb00076.x

[48] Higgins JA, Higbee DR, Donahoo WT, Brown IL, Bell ML, Bessesen DH. Resistant starch consumption promotes lipid oxidation. Journal of Nutrition and Metabolism. 2004;1(1):1-8. DOI: 10.1186/1743-7075-1-8

[49] Brown L, Rosner B, Willett WW, Sacks FM. Cholesterol-lowering effects of dietary fiber: a meta-analysis. The American journal of clinical nutrition. 1999 Jan 1;69(1):30-42.

50 https://www.health.harvard.edu/blog/fiber-full-eating-for-better-health-and-lower-cholesterol-2019062416819

[51] Pesta, Dominik H., and Varman T. Samuel. "A High-Protein Diet for Reducing Body Fat: Mechanisms and Possible Caveats - PMC." PubMed Central (PMC), 19 Nov. 2014, www.ncbi.nlm.nih.gov/pmc/articles/PMC4258944

[52] Pesta, Dominik H., and Varman T. Samuel. "A High-Protein

Diet for Reducing Body Fat: Mechanisms and Possible Caveats -
PMC." PubMed Central (PMC), 19 Nov. 2014,
www.ncbi.nlm.nih.gov/pmc/articles/PMC4258944

[53] Are Tannins a Double-Edged Sword in Biology and Health? -
ScienceDirect." Are Tannins a Double-Edged Sword in Biology
and Health? - ScienceDirect, 10 Jan. 1999,
www.sciencedirect.com/science/article/abs/pii/S092422449800
0284

[54] "Oxalate: Effect on Calcium Absorbability - PubMed."
PubMed, 1 Oct. 1989, pubmed.ncbi.nlm.nih.gov/2801588/

[55] "Antinutritional Properties of Plant Lectins - PubMed."
PubMed, 15 Sept. 2004, pubmed.ncbi.nlm.nih.gov/15302522/

[56] Nkhata, Smith G., et al. "Fermentation and Germination
Improve Nutritional Value of Cereals and Legumes through
Activation of Endogenous Enzymes - PMC." PubMed Central
(PMC), 16 Oct. 2018,
www.ncbi.nlm.nih.gov/pmc/articles/PMC6261201/

[57] Petroski, Weston, and Deanna M. Minich. "Is There Such a
Thing as 'Anti-Nutrients'? A Narrative Review of Perceived
Problematic Plant Compounds - PMC." PubMed Central (PMC),
24 Sept. 2020,
www.ncbi.nlm.nih.gov/pmc/articles/PMC7600777

[58] Malting is a process where grains are soaked and germinated.
They are then dried in shade and coarsely grinded.

[59] Finney, Patrick. 1982. "Effect of germination on cereal and
legume nutrient changes and food or feed value: a comprehensive

review." Chapter 12 in Recent Advances in Phytochemistry, Vol. 17. Mobilization of Reserves in Germination.

[60] Nkhata, Smith G., et al. "Fermentation and Germination Improve Nutritional Value of Cereals and Legumes through Activation of Endogenous Enzymes - PMC." PubMed Central (PMC), 16 Oct. 2018, www.ncbi.nlm.nih.gov/pmc/articles/PMC6261201

[61] Idowu, Anthony Temitope, et al. "Germination: An Alternative Source to Promote Phytonutrients in Edible Seeds | Food Quality and Safety | Oxford Academic." OUP Academic, 1 Aug. 2020, academic.oup.com/fqs/article/4/3/129/5685777

[62] Nandini, D. B., et al. "Sulforaphane in Broccoli: The Green Chemoprevention!! Role in Cancer Prevention and Therapy - PMC." PubMed Central (PMC), 9 Sept. 2020, www.ncbi.nlm.nih.gov/pmc/articles/PMC7802872/

[63] https://www.researchgate.net/publication/317306441_Why_do_millets_have_slower_starch_and_protein_digestibility_than_other_cereals

[64] Anitha, Seetha, et al. "Frontiers | A Systematic Review and Meta-Analysis of the Potential of Millets for Managing and Reducing the Risk of Developing Diabetes Mellitus." Frontiers, 1 Jan. 2001, www.frontiersin.org/articles/10.3389/fnut.2021.687428/full

[65] Cong Tang, Kashan Ahmed, Andreas Gille, Shun Lu,

Hermann-Josef Gröne, Sorin Tunaru & Stefan Offermanns
Loss of FFA2 and FFA3 increases insulin secretion and improves glucose tolerance in type 2 diabetes Nature Medicine, 2015

[66] Ostman, E. M. , Granfeldt, Y. , Persson, L. , & Bjorck, I. M. E. (2005). Vinegar supplementation lowers glucose and insulin responses and increases satiety after a bread meal in healthy subjects. European Journal of Clinical Nutrition, 59, 983–988. 10.1038/sj.ejcn.1602197

[67] Johnston CS, Buller AJ. Vinegar and peanut products as complementary foods to reduce postprandial glycemia. J Am Diet Assoc. 2005;105:1939–1942.

[68] "Vinegar Intake Reduces Body Weight, Body Fat Mass, and Serum Triglyceride Levels in Obese Japanese Subjects - PubMed." PubMed, 1 Aug. 2009, pubmed.ncbi.nlm.nih.gov/19661687.

[69] "Dietary Acetic Acid Reduces Serum Cholesterol and Triacylglycerols in Rats Fed a Cholesterol-Rich Diet - PubMed." PubMed, 1 May 2006, pubmed.ncbi.nlm.nih.gov/16611381

[70] Setorki, Mahbubeh, et al. "Acute Effects of Vinegar Intake on Some Biochemical Risk Factors of Atherosclerosis in Hypercholesterolemic Rabbits - PMC." PubMed Central (PMC), 28 Jan. 2010, www.ncbi.nlm.nih.gov/pmc/articles/PMC2837006

[71] "Apple Cider Vinegar Attenuates Oxidative Stress and Reduces the Risk of Obesity in High-Fat-Fed Male Wistar Rats - PubMed." PubMed, 1 Jan. 2018, pubmed.ncbi.nlm.nih.gov/29091513/

[72] Lee, Noo Ri, et al. "Application of Topical Acids Improves

Atopic Dermatitis in Murine Model by Enhancement of Skin Barrier Functions Regardless of the Origin of Acids - PMC." PubMed Central (PMC), 23 Nov. 2016, www.ncbi.nlm.nih.gov/pmc/articles/PMC5125949

[73] Food Groups and Risk of Coronary Heart Disease, Stroke and Heart Failure: A Systematic Review and Dose-Response Meta-Analysis of Prospective Studies - PubMed." PubMed, 1 Jan. 2019, pubmed.ncbi.nlm.nih.gov/29039970

[74] Associations of Processed Meat, Unprocessed Red Meat, Poultry, or Fish Intake With Incident Cardiovascular Disease and All-Cause Mortality - PubMed." PubMed, 1 Apr. 2020, pubmed.ncbi.nlm.nih.gov/32011623/

[75] Red Meat Intake and Risk of Coronary Heart Disease among US Men: Prospective Cohort Study - PubMed." PubMed, 2 Dec. 2020, pubmed.ncbi.nlm.nih.gov/33268459/

[76] Patterns of Red and Processed Meat Consumption and Risk for Cardiometabolic and Cancer Outcomes: A Systematic Review and Meta-Analysis of Cohort Studies - PubMed." PubMed, 19 Nov. 2019, pubmed.ncbi.nlm.nih.gov/31569217/

[77] Consumption of Meat, Fish, Dairy Products, and Eggs and Risk of Ischemic Heart Disease - PubMed." PubMed, 18 June 2019, pubmed.ncbi.nlm.nih.gov/31006335/

[78] "Dietary Patterns and Type 2 Diabetes: A Systematic Literature Review and Meta-Analysis of Prospective Studies - PubMed." PubMed, 1 June 2017, pubmed.ncbi.nlm.nih.gov/28424256/

[79] "Meat and Fish Intake and Type 2 Diabetes: Dose-Response

Meta-Analysis of Prospective Cohort Studies - PubMed."
PubMed, 1 Oct. 2020, pubmed.ncbi.nlm.nih.gov/32302686/

[80] "Food Groups and Risk of Type 2 Diabetes Mellitus: A
Systematic Review and Meta-Analysis of Prospective Studies -
PubMed."   PubMed,   1   May   2017,
pubmed.ncbi.nlm.nih.gov/28397016/

[81] "Replacing Red Meat and Processed Red Meat for White Meat,
Fish, Legumes or Eggs Is Associated with Lower Risk of
Incidence of Metabolic Syndrome - PubMed." PubMed, 1 Dec.
2016, pubmed.ncbi.nlm.nih.gov/27087650/

[82] "Diabetes Mellitus Associated with Processed and Unprocessed
Red Meat: An Overview - PubMed." PubMed, 1 Nov. 2016,
pubmed.ncbi.nlm.nih.gov/27309597/

[83] "Red Meat Consumption (Heme Iron Intake) and Risk for
Diabetes and Comorbidities? - PubMed." PubMed, 18 Sept. 2018,
pubmed.ncbi.nlm.nih.gov/30229313/

[84] "Meat and Fish Intake and Type 2 Diabetes: Dose-Response
Meta-Analysis of Prospective Cohort Studies - PubMed."
PubMed, 1 Oct. 2020, pubmed.ncbi.nlm.nih.gov/32302686/

[85]   https://www.who.int/news-room/questions-and-
answers/item/cancer-carcinogenicity-of-the-consumption-of-
red-meat-and-processed-meat

[86]   https://www.who.int/news-room/questions-and-answers/item/cancer-carcinogenicity-of-the-consumption-of-red-meat-and-processed-meat

[87]   Polycyclic Aromatic Hydrocarbons (PAHs) and Their Bioaccessibility in Meat: A Tool for Assessing Human Cancer Risk   -   PubMed."   PubMed,   1   Jan.   2016, pubmed.ncbi.nlm.nih.gov/26838201

[88] "Carcinogenicity of Consumption of Red and Processed Meat: What about Environmental Contaminants? - PubMed." PubMed, 1 Feb. 2016, pubmed.ncbi.nlm.nih.gov/26656511/

[89] Rizzo, Gianluca, et al. "Vitamin B12 among Vegetarians: Status, Assessment and Supplementation - PMC." PubMed Central (PMC),   29   Nov.   2016, www.ncbi.nlm.nih.gov/pmc/articles/PMC5188422/

[90] "Intake and Adequacy of the Vegan Diet. A Systematic Review of the Evidence - PubMed." PubMed, 1 May 2021, pubmed.ncbi.nlm.nih.gov/33341313/

[91] West, A. R., & Oates, P. S. (2008). Mechanisms of heme iron absorption: Current questions and controversies. World Journal of   Gastroenterology: WJG,   14(26),   4101–4110. doi:10.3748/wjg.14.4101

252

[92] Pawlak, Roman, et al. "Iron Status of Vegetarian Adults: A Review of Literature - PMC." PubMed Central (PMC), 16 Dec. 2016, www.ncbi.nlm.nih.gov/pmc/articles/PMC6367879/

[93] "The Effect of Vegetarian Diets on Iron Status in Adults: A Systematic Review and Meta-Analysis - PubMed." PubMed, 24 May 2018, pubmed.ncbi.nlm.nih.gov/27880062.

[94] Medicine (US) Panel on Micronutrients, Institute of. "Iron - Dietary Reference Intakes for Vitamin A, Vitamin K, Arsenic, Boron, Chromium, Copper, Iodine, Iron, Manganese, Molybdenum, Nickel, Silicon, Vanadium, and Zinc - NCBI Bookshelf." Iron - Dietary Reference Intakes for Vitamin A, Vitamin K, Arsenic, Boron, Chromium, Copper, Iodine, Iron, Manganese, Molybdenum, Nickel, Silicon, Vanadium, and Zinc - NCBI Bookshelf, 1 Jan. 2001, www.ncbi.nlm.nih.gov/books/NBK222309/

[95] Nebl, Josefine, et al. "Characterization, Dietary Habits and Nutritional Intake of Omnivorous, Lacto-Ovo Vegetarian and Vegan Runners – a Pilot Study - PMC." PubMed Central (PMC), 3 Dec. 2019, www.ncbi.nlm.nih.gov/pmc/articles/PMC7050782/

[96] "Seasonal Cycling in the Gut Microbiome of the Hadza Hunter-

Gatherers of Tanzania - PubMed." PubMed, 25 Aug. 2017, pubmed.ncbi.nlm.nih.gov/28839072/

97

https://www.sciencedaily.com/releases/2011/06/11061509451
4.htm

98

https://www.sciencedaily.com/releases/2011/06/11061509451
4.htm

99 "A Healthy Gastrointestinal Microbiome Is Dependent on Dietary Diversity - PubMed." PubMed, 5 Mar. 2016, pubmed.ncbi.nlm.nih.gov/27110483 and "Diversity, Compositional and Functional Differences between Gut Microbiota of Children and Adults - PubMed." PubMed, 23 Jan. 2020, pubmed.ncbi.nlm.nih.gov/31974429/ and D. Hills, Jr. Ronald, et al. "Gut Microbiome: Profound Implications for Diet and Disease - PMC." PubMed Central (PMC), 16 July 2019, www.ncbi.nlm.nih.gov/pmc/articles/PMC6682904

100 "Isolated Aerobic Exercise and Weight Loss: A Systematic Review and Meta-Analysis of Randomized Controlled Trials - PubMed." PubMed, 1 Aug. 2011, pubmed.ncbi.nlm.nih.gov/21787904.

[101] Changes in Energy Expenditure Resulting from Altered Body Weight | NEJM." Changes in Energy Expenditure Resulting from Altered Body Weight | NEJM, 10 Aug. 1995, www.nejm.org/doi/full/10.1056/nejm199503093321001

[102] Schulkin, Jay. "Evolutionary Basis of Human Running and Its Impact on Neural Function - PMC." PubMed Central (PMC), 11 July 2016, www.ncbi.nlm.nih.gov/pmc/articles/PMC4939291/

[103] Schulkin, Jay. "Evolutionary Basis of Human Running and Its Impact on Neural Function - PMC." PubMed Central (PMC), 11 July 2016, www.ncbi.nlm.nih.gov/pmc/articles/PMC4939291/

104 A Neuroimaging Investigation of the Association between Aerobic Fitness, Hippocampal Volume, and Memory Performance in Preadolescent Children - PubMed." PubMed, 28 Oct. 2010, pubmed.ncbi.nlm.nih.gov/20735996/

105 "Aerobic Fitness Is Associated with Hippocampal Volume in Elderly Humans - PubMed." PubMed, 1 Oct. 2009, pubmed.ncbi.nlm.nih.gov/19123237/

106 Relationship between Exercise Capacity and Brain Size in Mammals - PubMed." PubMed, 1 Jan. 2011, pubmed.ncbi.nlm.nih.gov/21731619

107 Relationship between Exercise Capacity and Brain Size in Mammals - PubMed." PubMed, 1 Jan. 2011, pubmed.ncbi.nlm.nih.gov/21731619

108 Schusdziarra, Volker, et al. "Impact of Breakfast on Daily Energy Intake - an Analysis of Absolute versus Relative Breakfast Calories - Nutrition Journal." BioMed Central, 17 Jan. 2011, nutritionj.biomedcentral.com/articles/10.1186/1475-2891-10-5.

109 Sievert, Katherine, et al. "Effect of Breakfast on Weight and Energy Intake: Systematic Review and Meta-Analysis of Randomised Controlled Trials | The BMJ." The BMJ, 1 Jan. 2019, www.bmj.com/content/364/bmj.l42

110 Anton, Stephen D., et al. "Flipping the Metabolic Switch: Understanding and Applying Health Benefits of Fasting - PMC." PubMed Central (PMC), 31 Oct. 2017, www.ncbi.nlm.nih.gov/pmc/articles/PMC5783752/

111 Ho, K. Y., et al. "Fasting Enhances Growth Hormone Secretion and Amplifies the Complex Rhythms of Growth Hormone Secretion in Man. - PMC." PubMed Central (PMC), www.ncbi.nlm.nih.gov/pmc/articles/PMC329619. Accessed 11

112 "Intermittent Fasting vs Daily Calorie Restriction for Type 2 Diabetes Prevention: A Review of Human Findings." Intermittent Fasting vs Daily Calorie Restriction for Type 2 Diabetes Prevention: A Review of Human Findings - ScienceDirect, 12 June   2014, www.sciencedirect.com/science/article/abs/pii/S193152441400200X

113 Harvie, M. N., et al. "The Effects of Intermittent or Continuous Energy Restriction on Weight Loss and Metabolic Disease Risk Markers: A Randomized Trial in Young Overweight Women - International Journal of Obesity." Nature, 5 Oct. 2010, www.nature.com/articles/ijo2010171

114 "Insulin Levels, Hunger, and Food Intake: An Example of Feedback Loops in Body Weight Regulation - PubMed." PubMed, 1 Jan. 1985, pubmed.ncbi.nlm.nih.gov/3894001/

115 "Early Time-Restricted Feeding Reduces Appetite and Increases Fat Oxidation But Does Not Affect Energy Expenditure in Humans - PubMed." PubMed, 1 Aug. 2019, pubmed.ncbi.nlm.nih.gov/31339000/

116 "Changes in Hunger and Fullness in Relation to Gut Peptides

before and after 8 Weeks of Alternate Day Fasting - PubMed."
PubMed, 1 Dec. 2016, pubmed.ncbi.nlm.nih.gov/27062219/

117 Anton, Stephen D., et al. "Flipping the Metabolic Switch:
Understanding and Applying Health Benefits of Fasting - PMC."
PubMed Central (PMC), 31 Oct. 2017,
www.ncbi.nlm.nih.gov/pmc/articles/PMC5783752/

118 "Effect of Alternate-Day Fasting on Weight Loss, Weight
Maintenance, and Cardioprotection Among Metabolically
Healthy Obese Adults: A Randomized Clinical Trial - PubMed."
PubMed, 1 July 2017, pubmed.ncbi.nlm.nih.gov/28459931/

119 "Effects of Intermittent Fasting on Body Composition and
Clinical Health Markers in Humans - PubMed." PubMed, 1 Oct.
2015, pubmed.ncbi.nlm.nih.gov/26374764

120 "Effects of 4- and 6-h Time-Restricted Feeding on Weight
and Cardiometabolic Health: A Randomized Controlled Trial in
Adults with Obesity - PubMed." PubMed, 1 Sept. 2020,
pubmed.ncbi.nlm.nih.gov/32673591

121 "A Randomised Controlled Trial of the 5:2 Diet - PubMed."
PubMed, 17 Nov. 2021, pubmed.ncbi.nlm.nih.gov/34788298

122 "Intermittent Fasting vs Daily Calorie Restriction for Type 2

Diabetes Prevention: A Review of Human Findings." Intermittent Fasting vs Daily Calorie Restriction for Type 2 Diabetes Prevention: A Review of Human Findings - ScienceDirect, 12 June 2014, www.sciencedirect.com/science/article/abs/pii/S193152441400 200X

123 Carroll, Paul V., et al. "Growth Hormone Deficiency in Adulthood and the Effects of Growth Hormone Replacement: A Review | The Journal of Clinical Endocrinology and Metabolism | Oxford Academic." OUP Academic, 1 Feb. 1998, academic.oup.com/jcem/article/83/2/382/2865179

124 "Growth Hormone Improves Body Composition, Fat Utilization, Physical Strength and Agility, and Growth in Prader-Willi Syndrome: A Controlled Study - PubMed." PubMed, 1 Feb. 1999, pubmed.ncbi.nlm.nih.gov/9931532/

125 "Growth Hormone Improves Body Composition, Fat Utilization, Physical Strength and Agility, and Growth in Prader-Willi Syndrome: A Controlled Study - PubMed." PubMed, 1 Feb. 1999, pubmed.ncbi.nlm.nih.gov/9931532/

126 "Massive Weight Loss Restores 24-Hour Growth Hormone Release Profiles and Serum Insulin-like Growth Factor-I Levels in Obese Subjects - PubMed." PubMed, 1 Apr. 1995,

pubmed.ncbi.nlm.nih.gov/7536210/

127 "Elevated Insulin Levels Contribute to the Reduced Growth Hormone (GH) Response to GH-Releasing Hormone in Obese Subjects - PubMed." PubMed, 1 Sept. 1999, pubmed.ncbi.nlm.nih.gov/10484056/

128 "Fasting Enhances Growth Hormone Secretion and Amplifies the Complex Rhythms of Growth Hormone Secretion in Man - PubMed." PubMed, 1 Apr. 1988, pubmed.ncbi.nlm.nih.gov/3127426/

129 Augmented Growth Hormone (GH) Secretory Burst Frequency and Amplitude Mediate Enhanced GH Secretion during a Two-Day Fast in Normal Men - PubMed." PubMed, 1 Apr. 1992, pubmed.ncbi.nlm.nih.gov/1548337

130 Chung, Ki Wung, and Hae Young Chung. "The Effects of Calorie Restriction on Autophagy: Role on Aging Intervention - PMC." PubMed Central (PMC), 2 Dec. 2019, www.ncbi.nlm.nih.gov/pmc/articles/PMC6950580.

131 "The Effect of Fasting or Calorie Restriction on Autophagy Induction: A Review of the Literature - PubMed." PubMed, 1 Nov. 2018, pubmed.ncbi.nlm.nih.gov/30172870/

132 Antunes, Fernanda, et al. "Autophagy and Intermittent Fasting: The Connection for Cancer Therapy? - PMC." PubMed Central (PMC), 27 Nov. 2018, www.ncbi.nlm.nih.gov/pmc/articles/PMC6257056

133 Longo, Valter D., and Mark P. Mattson. "Fasting: Molecular Mechanisms and Clinical Applications - PMC." PubMed Central (PMC), 16 Jan. 2014, www.ncbi.nlm.nih.gov/pmc/articles/PMC3946160

134 Caffeine, Coffee, and Appetite Control: A Review - PubMed." PubMed, 1 Dec. 2017, pubmed.ncbi.nlm.nih.gov/28446037

135 "The Growing Problem of Obesity in Dogs and Cats - PubMed." PubMed, 1 July 2006, pubmed.ncbi.nlm.nih.gov/16772464/

136 Chusyd, Daniella E., et al. "Adiposity and Reproductive Cycling Status in Zoo African Elephants - PMC." PubMed Central (PMC), www.ncbi.nlm.nih.gov/pmc/articles/PMC5744898

137 "The Importance of Habits in Eating Behaviour. An Overview and Recommendations for Future Research - PubMed." PubMed, 1 Dec. 2011, pubmed.ncbi.nlm.nih.gov/21816186

138 PMC, Europe. "Europe PMC." Europe PMC, europepmc.org/article/MED/14599286.

139 "Situational Effects on Meal Intake: A Comparison of Eating Alone and Eating with Others - ScienceDirect." Situational Effects on Meal Intake: A Comparison of Eating Alone and Eating with Others - ScienceDirect, 6 June 2006, www.sciencedirect.com/science/article/abs/pii/S003193840600 1879

140 Neary, Nicola, and Lynnette Nieman. "Adrenal Insufficiency-Etiology, Diagnosis and Treatment - PMC." PubMed Central (PMC), www.ncbi.nlm.nih.gov/pmc/articles/PMC2928659/

141 Adam, Tanja C., et al. "Cortisol Is Negatively Associated with Insulin Sensitivity in Overweight Latino Youth - PMC." PubMed Central (PMC), 21 July 2010, www.ncbi.nlm.nih.gov/pmc/articles/PMC3050109/

142 An in Vivo and in Vitro Study of the Mechanism of Prednisone-Induced Insulin Resistance in Healthy Subjects - PubMed." PubMed, 1 Nov. 1983, pubmed.ncbi.nlm.nih.gov/6355186

143 "Stress Cortisol Connection." Stress Cortisol Connection, www.unm.edu/~lkravitz/Article%20folder/stresscortisol.html

144 https://journals.lww.com/psychosomaticmedicine/Abstract/20 00/09000/Stress_and_Body_Shape__Stress_Induced_Cortisol.5 .aspx

145 Stress May Add Bite to Appetite in Women: A Laboratory Study of Stress-Induced Cortisol and Eating Behavior - PubMed." PubMed, 1 Jan. 2001, pubmed.ncbi.nlm.nih.gov/11070333/

146 Appetite-Regulating Hormones Cortisol and Peptide YY Are Associated with Disordered Eating Psychopathology, Independent of Body Mass Index - PubMed." PubMed, 1 Feb. 2011, pubmed.ncbi.nlm.nih.gov/21098684

147 Neary, Nicola, and Lynnette Nieman. "Adrenal Insufficiency-Etiology, Diagnosis and Treatment - PMC." PubMed Central (PMC), www.ncbi.nlm.nih.gov/pmc/articles/PMC2928659/

148 Audrain-McGovern, J., and NL Benowitz. "Cigarette Smoking, Nicotine, and Body Weight - PMC." PubMed Central (PMC), 1 June 2011, www.ncbi.nlm.nih.gov/pmc/articles/PMC3195407/

Printed in Great Britain
by Amazon